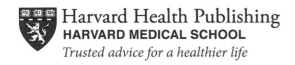

Harvard Health Publishing
HARVARD MEDICAL SCHOOL
Trusted advice for a healthier life

D0907282

Dear Reader,

Of your five senses, which one are you most afraid of losing? If you're like most people, the answer is your ability to see. Despite this, many people are not conscientious about caring for their eyes and often neglect to visit an ophthalmologist for routine eye exams as they get older.

Like the rest of your body, your eyes naturally change throughout your life. These changes occur gradually and become apparent in later years, as the structures in and around your eyes become less efficient. For most people, the first sign is presbyopia, the deterioration of close-up vision. Luckily, this problem can be managed with reading glasses or progressive lenses.

However, more serious age-related eye problems can cause vision loss or visual distortion that glasses can't fix. More than seven million adults ages 65 and over in the United States have significant vision loss, meaning they can't see clearly, even with the aid of glasses or contact lenses. The vast majority of them weren't born with vision impairment. They lost their sight to diseases like macular degeneration, glaucoma, and diabetes. Over the next 30 years, the number of blind or visually impaired Americans is expected to more than double as the baby boomer generation ages. For most of these eye diseases, early detection and treatment can prevent or curb vision loss.

This report covers normal age-related conditions, such as presbyopia, as well as the four eye diseases that pose the greatest threats to vision after age 40: cataracts, glaucoma, age-related macular degeneration, and diabetic retinopathy. It also describes other common eye disorders, including dry eye, flashes and floaters, retinal detachment, and eyelid problems such as drooping upper or lower lids.

You'll learn why you should have regular eye exams, especially if you have diabetes or a family history of glaucoma or age-related macular degeneration; how to recognize the risk factors and symptoms of specific eye diseases; and what steps you can take to prevent or treat them before your vision deteriorates further. You'll learn about the latest advances in cataract surgery, as well as cutting-edge treatments for age-related macular degeneration. This report also provides specific information about what you can do to protect your eyes—and your vision—throughout your lifetime.

Sincerely,

Laura Fine, M.D.
Medical Editor

Jeffrey Heier, M.D.
Medical Editor

Harvard Health Publishing | Harvard Medical School | 4 Blackfan Circle, 4th Floor | Boston, MA 02115

How the eye works

The eye is often compared to a camera, but in truth, the organ of sight is far more complex and efficient than even the most sophisticated and expensive camera. Not only does the eye continuously focus and snap pictures, but it also works with the brain and nervous system to process every image that crosses your line of sight, providing you with the visual information you need to do everything from drive a car to sketch a picture. And though you can replace even the priciest camera, it would be virtually impossible to precisely replicate the sophisticated layers of machinery that control the human eye and connect it to the brain.

That said, your vision will likely change over your lifetime. Knowing the basics of eye anatomy can help you understand any changes that occur, whether they stem from the normal aging process or an eye disease.

Protection from without

Despite its reputation as a delicate organ, the eye is remarkably resilient and hardy, engineered by nature to last from infancy through old age. It sits in a bony, protective socket of the skull, called the orbit, and is surrounded by a cushiony layer of fibrous tissue, fat, and a set of six muscles (extraocular muscles) that regulate its movements (see Figure 1, above right).

The eyeball itself is sturdy, too. Its outer surface (approximately 1 millimeter thick) is made of tough collagen. You see it in the visible part of the eyeball as both the sclera (the white part) and the cornea, a clear, dome-like window at the front of the eye that allows light to enter.

Eyelids and eyelashes provide additional protection, acting like windshield wipers to constantly brush and blink away dust and debris that might otherwise blow into the eye. Tears from the lacrimal gland, located behind the upper lid, course over the surface of the eye and keep it lubricated, nourished, and clear of foreign matter.

Figure 1: Eye anatomy: The outside view

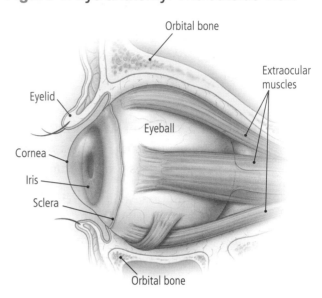

The eyeball is surrounded by ligaments, fat, and muscles and rests in a protective, bony socket called the orbit. Six extraocular muscles control the eyeball's movement. The cornea (a tough, transparent dome that helps focus light) and the sclera (the white portion of the eye) protect the interior of the eye.

Less obvious protection comes from the conjunctiva—a thin, transparent membrane that lines the inner surfaces of the eyelids and the front portion of the sclera. The conjunctiva is so sensitive that when it detects a foreign body, it automatically triggers a protective reaction, such as tearing or blinking.

An exquisite structure within

The inner architecture of the eye is complex, with more than a dozen interconnected parts that work together. Some of these structures are quite familiar—others, less so.

The eye consists of two major compartments—the front (including the lens, iris, cornea, and aqueous humor) and the back (the rear two-thirds of the eyeball, including the retina and a large cavity filled with

THE AGING EYE
SPECIAL HEALTH REPORT

Medical Editors
Laura C. Fine, MD
Clinical Instructor in Ophthalmology,
Harvard Medical School
Glaucoma and Cataract Specialist,
Ophthalmic Consultants of Boston
President, New England Ophthalmological
Society

Jeffrey S. Heier, MD
Clinical Instructor in Ophthalmology,
Harvard Medical School
Co-President and Medical Director,
Ophthalmic Consultants of Boston

Executive Editor
Anne Underwood

Writer   **Copy Editor**
Stephanie Watson   Robin Netherton

Production/Design Manager
Susan Dellenbaugh

Illustrators
Harriet Greenfield, Scott Leighton

Published by Harvard Medical School
David Roberts, MD, *Dean for External Education*
Urmila R. Parlikar, *Associate Director, Digital*
Health Products

IN ASSOCIATION WITH

Belvoir Media Group, LLC, 535 Connecticut Avenue, Norwalk, CT 06854-1713. Robert Englander, Chairman and CEO; Timothy H. Cole, Executive Vice President, Belvoir Editorial Director; Philip L. Penny, Chief Operating Officer; Greg King, Executive Vice President, Marketing Director; Ron Goldberg, Chief Financial Officer; Tom Canfield, Vice President, Circulation.

Website
For the latest information and most up-to-date publication list, visit us online at www.health.harvard.edu.

Customer Service
For all subscription questions or problems (rates, subscribing, address changes, billing problems), email HarvardProd@StrategicFulfillment.com, call 877-649-9457 (toll-free), or write to Harvard Health Publishing, P.O. Box 9308, Big Sandy, TX 75755-9308.

Ordering Special Health Reports
Harvard Medical School publishes Special Health Reports on a wide range of topics. To order copies of this or other reports, please see the instructions at the back of this report, or go to our website: www.health.harvard.edu.

For Licensing, Bulk Rates, or Corporate Sales
email HHP_licensing@hms.harvard.edu,
or visit www.content.health.harvard.edu.

ISBN 978-1-61401-201-6

Contents

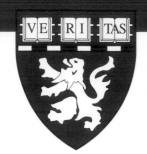

A HARVARD MEDICAL SCHOOL
SPECIAL HEALTH REPORT

The Aging Eye

Preventing and treating eye disease

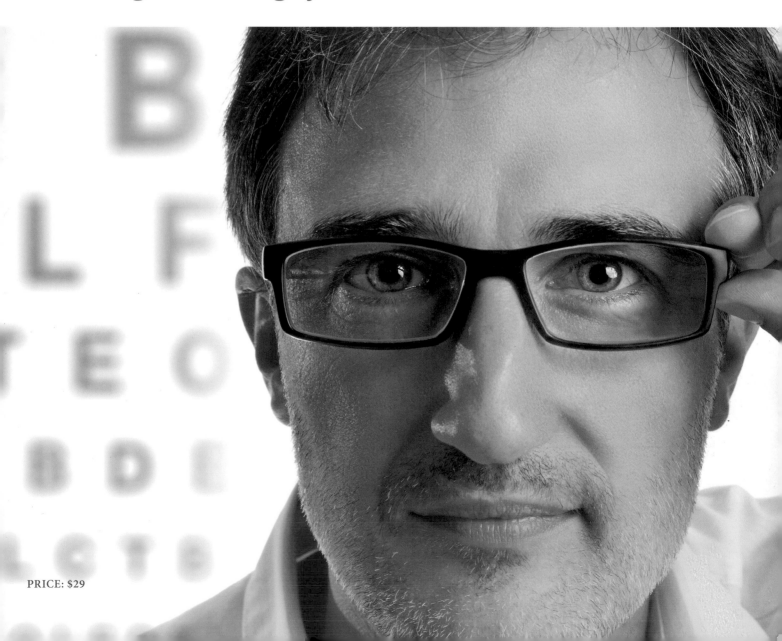

PRICE: $29

vitreous humor; see Figure 2, at right). Structures in both sections are essential for sight.

In the front compartment, the iris is the pigmented section that gives your eye its color, which might be blue, green, brown, or hazel. Like an automatic camera, which adjusts the size of its aperture (opening) to the available light, the iris controls how much light enters the eye through the pupil—the black hole at the center of the iris. The involuntary muscles of the iris open to allow more light to enter the pupil in dim light, and close to make the pupil smaller in bright light. A good example of the eye's adaptation is the change that occurs when you walk into sunlight after sitting in a dark movie theater. Even subtle alterations in light prompt a response from the eye, and the iris muscles are continually adjusting to the environment.

Just behind the pupil and iris is the lens. The purpose of the lens is to focus light rays on the retina, the thin, light-sensitive inner layer at the rear of the eye. Tiny ciliary muscles attached to the lens enable it to alter its shape so the eye can focus on objects at varying distances. When you look at a tree far away, the muscles cause the lens to flatten. But shift your gaze to something close, such as a computer screen, and the muscles contract, which makes the lens thicker and more curved in the middle. The ability of the lens to adjust its focus is called accommodation.

The anterior chamber is an area between the cornea and the iris (see Figure 2, above right). It is filled

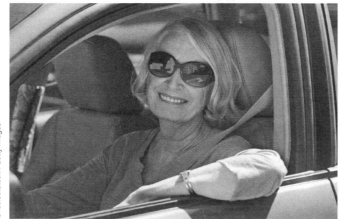

The muscles of the iris (the colored part of your eye) are continually adjusting to allow the right amount of light to enter the eye. Similarly, the lens is continually adjusting its focus.

Figure 2: Eye anatomy: The inside story

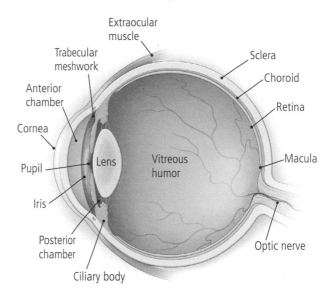

Rays of light pass through the cornea, the anterior chamber, and then the lens, which focuses images. The lens is nourished by the aqueous humor, a clear, watery solution that circulates from the posterior chamber into the anterior chamber and helps maintain normal pressure. Light reaches the retina after it passes from the lens through the vitreous humor, a clear gel that fills most of the eyeball. The retina has light-sensitive cells that capture images, which are then sent to the brain via the optic nerve. At the retina's center is the macula, a small region that provides sharp, central vision.

with a clear liquid called aqueous humor, which nourishes the lens and removes wastes. The aqueous humor flows into this region from the posterior chamber—the area between the iris and the lens. It flows out through the trabecular meshwork and Schlemm's canal, a circular drainage system located where the clear cornea, white sclera, and colored iris meet. In a healthy eye, this circulation constantly drains and resupplies the aqueous humor, maintaining a balance of fluid in the two chambers.

The ciliary body behind the iris produces the aqueous humor. It also contains the ciliary muscles, which help the lens change shape as your eye focuses.

In the back of the eyeball are other crucial structures. The retina is a mass of nerve cells and fibers where images are captured and recorded, much like the film in an old-fashioned camera. Within the retina are light-sensitive cells called photoreceptors, including about 120 million rods and six million cones—specialized cells made up of chemicals that react to different wavelengths of light. Each performs a specific function:

- The cones perceive color and are responsible for fine detail in the center of vision. They enable you to read words on a page and to recognize a familiar face from across the room. Cones are most active in bright light.
- The rods do not perceive color, but rather light, shadow, and motion. They are most sensitive in the dark, which explains why it is hard to detect colors and fine details in the dark. They are found throughout the retina, but most are in the periphery.

The macula, the tiny part of the retina that gives you sharp central vision, is where most of the cones are located. But the best vision—for reading or detailed work—comes from the fovea, which is at the center of the macula. The rest of the retina delivers peripheral (side) vision, which is less sharply focused.

The choroid is sandwiched between the sclera and retina in the rear of the eye. This membrane is packed with blood vessels that carry oxygen and other nourishment to the outer part of the retina.

The images striking the retina travel to the brain via the optic nerve, which relays information about the size, shape, color, and distance of the objects you see.

Most of these structures are located near the outer layer of the eyeball, in either the front or back. But the inner chamber of the eye is not empty. Rather, it is filled with vitreous humor. Unlike aqueous humor, which is a liquid, the vitreous humor is a clear, stable gel that looks like raw egg white. It gives shape to the eye and provides a pathway for light coming through the lens to the retina.

The art of seeing

Sight is not fully developed at birth; the brain and eyes have to learn to work together in the first months of life. Once sight is well developed, the eyes and brain team up to provide virtually instantaneous visual information.

To illustrate this process, imagine that you're sightseeing in Washington, D.C., and you've stopped to look at the blooming cherry trees. What you are actually seeing is the light reflected off the trees. Some light must be present in order for you to see them.

Light rays thrown off the surfaces of the trees hit your cornea, which refracts, or bends, them inward so they pass into the eye to the lens. The lens bends the light rays further to produce a clear image and projects them onto the retina as a flat, upside-down image.

The retina absorbs the light and turns it into electrical energy, which the optic nerve then conveys to the visual area of the brain. Data about the trees—their size, shape, color, and position—are sent along the optic nerve as impulses, a sort of neurologic code that the brain deciphers. Although the image is upside down on the retina, the brain automatically turns it right side up.

Although it is possible to see with only one eye, you generally rely on binocular vision—vision with both eyes—for depth perception. You get a three-dimensional view of the trees because your brain

Figure 3: Normal vision

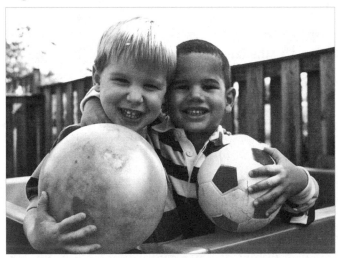

The National Eye Institute created a series of photos to demonstrate how different eye problems affect vision. The photo above shows how a person with normal vision would see these two boys while standing 20 feet away from them. In this report, you'll find examples of how people with cataracts, glaucoma, age-related macular degeneration, and diabetic retinopathy would see the same boys.
Photo courtesy of the National Eye Institute.

interprets what your two eyes see (each with a slightly different perspective) as a single image. (People who are blind in one eye get their depth perception from clues, such as relative size of objects and motion parallax—perceiving objects closer to themselves as moving faster than objects farther away.)

In addition, the external muscles of your eyes are synchronized to keep your eyes aligned and to coordinate their movement. If a child were to suddenly run by, you could instantly shift your gaze without giving it a thought.

Why aging may cause problems

Just as hair turns gray and skin sags with age, the eyes, too, undergo changes as you grow older. Although many of these changes are part of the normal aging process, some set the stage for more serious eye problems.

As your eyes age, your eyelid muscles weaken, and skin becomes thinner and more flaccid. This can cause the upper lid to droop or the lower lid to sag. Eyelashes and eyebrows may lose their lushness and thin out considerably.

Tear production also drops with age. In addition, the oily film that protects tears from evaporating decreases as lubricating glands in the conjunctiva and lids reduce their output. These changes can lead to a buildup of sticky mucus or can dry out the cornea, causing irritation or an uncomfortable, gritty sensation in the eye, as well as fluctuations in vision.

The conjunctiva turns thinner and more fragile with age and takes on a yellowish tinge from an increase in elastin fibers. The white of your eye (the sclera) also assumes a yellow hue from a collection of lipid, or fat, deposits. Calcium may deposit in the sclera, leading to grayish translucent patches. The exposed conjunctiva between the lids begins to degenerate, and the cornea can develop an opaque white ring around its edge.

With time, the lens hardens and loses its elasticity. This makes it more difficult to focus on near objects, a common condition called presbyopia. You might find that your night vision grows poorer. A decrease in pupil size and photoreceptor function

Warning signs that warrant a doctor visit

See an ophthalmologist if you experience any of the following symptoms or problems with your eyes:

- Change in iris color
- Crossed eyes
- Dark spot in the center of your field of vision
- Difficulty focusing on near or distant objects
- Double vision
- Dry eyes with itching or burning
- Episodes of cloudy vision
- Excess discharge or tearing
- Eye pain
- Floaters or flashes
- Growing bump on the eyelid
- Halos (colored circles around lights) or glare
- Hazy or blurred vision
- Inability to close your eyelid
- Loss of peripheral vision
- Redness in or around the eye
- Spots in your field of vision
- Sudden loss of vision
- Trouble adjusting to dark rooms
- Unusual sensitivity to light or glare
- Veil obstructing vision
- Wavy or crooked appearance to straight lines

with age also makes it harder for your eyes to adapt to the dark. These changes usually occur simultaneously in both eyes.

More serious age-related problems

Growing older contributes to a number of other eye changes that need to be monitored and treated (see "Warning signs that warrant a doctor visit," above). Following are the most common ones, all of which are covered at length later in this report. In addition, certain medications you take can affect your eyes (see "Medications that can affect your eyes," page 6).

Cataract. This clouding of the lens usually develops slowly over many years. You may not notice the cloudiness until it blocks your central line of sight and impairs your vision.

Glaucoma. Over time, the anterior chamber in each eye may become shallower in certain people—those who have small eyes and are farsighted, for example. The narrowing can lead to a blockage in the aqueous humor drainage system near the iris. The

▶ Medications that can affect your eyes

Talk to your eye doctor about the medications you take for other conditions, because they circulate through your entire body and can affect your eyes. For example:

- **Amiodarone** (Cordarone, Pacerone) for an irregular heart rhythm can cause deposits called verticillata to form on the cornea.

- **Antihistamines** used to treat allergies can worsen closed-angle glaucoma (see page 30).

- **Antipsychotic drugs** such as chlorpromazine (Thorazine) and thioridazine (Mellaril) used to treat schizophrenia and other mental health issues can damage your retina.

- **Bisphosphonates** such as alendronate (Fosamax) and risedronate (Actonel) used to prevent bone loss in postmenopausal women can cause eye inflammation (uveitis and scleritis).

- **Corticosteroids** such as prednisone (Deltasone) for arthritis and other ailments can lead to cataracts and increased pressure in the eye with long-term use.

- **Hydroxychloroquine** (Plaquenil) used to prevent malaria and treat rheumatoid arthritis can cause retinal damage.

- **Tamsulosin** (Flomax), which treats prostate enlargement in men, can increase your risks in cataract surgery.

- **Topiramate** (Topamax) for treating epilepsy and migraine headaches can cause closed-angle glaucoma.

---

resulting fluid backup may lead to a sudden or rapid rise in pressure inside the eye that damages the optic nerve, a condition known as closed-angle glaucoma. Left untreated, it can cause blindness.

Another form of glaucoma, called open-angle glaucoma, occurs when pressure builds up gradually in the eye because of a different problem: a slower outflow of aqueous humor through the trabecular meshwork. As in closed-angle glaucoma, the resulting buildup of pressure inside the eye can damage the optic nerve, if left untreated.

Age-related macular degeneration. The aging retina thins and may grow less sensitive to light because of cell loss, a reduced blood supply, or degeneration. The macula is especially prone to deteriora-tion. Age-related macular degeneration is a serious disease that can steal a person's central vision, making it difficult to read, write, or drive a car.

Diabetic retinopathy. Diabetes is a disease in which the body either doesn't produce enough insulin or doesn't use it effectively. Insulin normally moves sugar from the blood to the cells for energy. Without it, sugar builds up in the bloodstream and can damage blood vessels and organs throughout the body—including the eyes. Diabetic retinopathy occurs when blood vessels that feed the retina leak, leading to retinal swelling. When left untreated over time, this condition can lead to blindness.

Many treatments are available for the above conditions to preserve vision. ◆

Common changes in the aging eye

Many people will never have to deal with serious eye disease. But nearly everyone will eventually experience some age-related changes in vision, and in the function and structure of different parts of their eyes, from front to back.

General ophthalmologists are able to treat many of these issues. However, in some situations involving problems with the eyelids, tear drainage, or skin cancer, you may be referred to an oculoplastic specialist—a doctor with advanced training in plastic and reconstructive surgery of the eyelid and surrounding tissues (see "Your eye professionals," page 18). For problems with the cornea, retina, or optic nerve, you may be referred to specialists in these fields.

Presbyopia: Hello, reading glasses

You might have already noticed that you have to hold your menu at arm's length to read it, especially in a dimly lit restaurant. Presbyopia—from the Greek words for "old sight"—is a reduction in the eye's ability to focus. It may start as early as your late 30s, but it typically develops in the 40s and 50s and eventually affects everyone. Presbyopia occurs when the aging lens becomes more rigid and less efficient at bending to accommodate changes in focus. An accompanying lag in the function of the ciliary muscles—the ring of muscles that helps the lens focus near or far—contributes to the difficulty in seeing small print.

Blurred close vision that leaves eyes tired and strained is an early hint that you've developed pres-

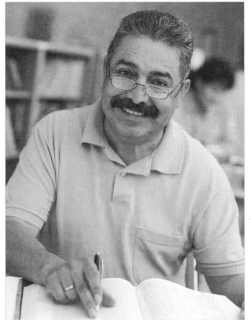

Whether your eyesight was good or bad in your youth, you will eventually develop presbyopia. The most common remedy is reading glasses

byopia. After reading or doing other detail work, you may find it hard to see distant objects clearly. The problem may be more pronounced when you try to read in poor light, or in the evening when you are tired. The condition occurs regardless of whether you are nearsighted, farsighted, or astigmatic (see Figure 4, page 9). However, presbyopia often affects farsighted people at a younger age than nearsighted people. If you're nearsighted, you may be able to overcome presbyopia at first by taking off your glasses to read. Eventually, as your presbyopia worsens and the lens of your eye becomes stiffer, you may need new corrective lenses.

The most common remedy for presbyopia is reading glasses. Prescription glasses provide the greatest precision, but many drugstores and supermarkets carry inexpensive reading glasses that may work well for you. Have your ophthalmologist perform an eye exam before you purchase a pair of reading glasses, so you'll know which strength to buy.

If you already wear glasses, you might consider bifocals, trifocals, or progressive lenses, which combine several levels of adjustment to correct both distance and close-up vision problems. Some people use two pairs of glasses—one for distance and one for close work.

If you wear contact lenses, multifocal contact lenses that combine several levels of adjustment (bifocal, trifocal, or progressive lenses) are available. Or you can get one prescription contact lens that corrects the vision in one eye for reading, and another lens that corrects for distance—a technique called monovision (see "Surgical monovision," below).

Whichever type of lens you choose, you may need to update your prescription often, because presbyopia becomes worse with age. It should finally stabilize between ages 60 and 65.

Surgical monovision. Another option for people ages 40 to 60 who have presbyopia but otherwise healthy eyes is to surgically correct one eye for close-up vision, leaving the other for distance vision. Monovision doesn't fix the stiffened lenses that cause presbyopia, but it can eliminate the need for bifocals or multiple sets of glasses, and it may even enable you to read without glasses. However, one eye will be slightly sharper than the other at specific distances, which could affect your depth perception.

Doctors use various procedures to make the correction. Laser surgery techniques include laser-assisted in situ keratomileusis (LASIK), photorefractive keratectomy (PRK), and laser thermal keratoplasty (LTK), each of which reshapes the cornea or the area around it. (The technique used depends on your particular circumstances.) If you choose laser surgery and you still have good distance vision, the surgeon will correct one eye so you can see up close, leaving the other eye with your natural ability to see far. If you're both myopic and presbyopic, the doctor can correct your nondominant eye for near vision and your dominant eye for distance. It may take several surgeries to get the desired result, and the results may not last.

Another technique used for monovision is conductive keratoplasty (CK). This method is similar to laser surgery, but instead of a laser, it uses short bursts of radio waves to shrink and reshape the cornea. One limitation is that it can take a few months before you experience the full benefits. There is also a slight risk that CK may cause astigmatism.

Monovision isn't for everyone. It is vital that your eyes be healthy and free from other eye defects, such as cataracts, glaucoma, or corneal problems. Some people find it too difficult to adjust to different focusing abilities in each eye. If you're considering this surgery, try monovision with contact lenses first, to see whether you can adjust.

Refractive lens exchange (clear lens extraction). Replacing a still-healthy natural lens—one that hasn't been clouded by a cataract—is controversial and isn't often done, but some ophthalmologists will replace the clear natural lenses in middle-aged or older people who have refractive vision errors like presbyopia and hyperopia (see Figure 4, page 9), but who aren't candidates for LASIK corrective surgery.

Keep two things in mind before undergoing refractive lens exchange surgery. First, it is not approved by the FDA and will not be covered by insurance unless you need the lens replacement to treat cataracts. (The cost can range from $2,500 to $4,500 for each eye.) Replacement lenses that correct for astigmatism or presbyopia carry an additional cost. Second, many ophthalmologists are reluctant to perform this procedure in people without cataracts because of risks like retinal detachment and vision loss, and because they don't have good data on its long-term safety and effectiveness.

Phakic intraocular lenses. These surgically implanted lenses may be an alternative to LASIK for correcting nearsightedness, farsightedness, or astigmatism. Unlike cataract surgery, which replaces your natural lens, this procedure involves placing an additional lens either between the cornea and the iris or just behind the iris, without removing your own lens. The phakic lens bends light rays to focus them more precisely on your retina. Two FDA-approved phakic lenses are available—Verisyse and Visian Implantable Collamer Lens. However, a number of risks are associated with phakic lenses, including possible vision loss or vision problems such as halos, glare, or double vision. The lenses also increase your risk of developing glaucoma or cataracts.

Double vision

When your eyes are working correctly, you should see images clearly. But sometimes, you might see not one, but two of the same image. This is called double vision, or diplopia.

Double vision can occur with one eye open (monocular diplopia), usually because of a focusing problem with the eye. More often, you'll see double with both eyes open (binocular diplopia), which occurs when the eyes are misaligned.

Causes of double vision include the following:

- astigmatism (see Figure 4, below)
- cataracts
- Graves' or thyroid disease
- a problem with the shape of the cornea
- multiple sclerosis
- myasthenia gravis (an autoimmune disease that affects the muscles)
- an aneurysm, tumor, or another growth that presses on a nerve
- paralysis of nerves controlling muscles that move the eye
- stroke
- swelling or infection of the eye.

Any double vision warrants a visit to an ophthalmologist for testing. The ophthalmologist will assess whether the double vision is a byproduct of an underlying condition, such as thyroid disease, in which case you will also need to have that condition treated. Your ophthalmologist may order additional testing, including imaging studies such as an MRI, to rule out nervous system (neurologic) causes of the double vision. Treatment options depend on the nature of the problem and might include corrective lenses, prism glasses (which bend the light that shines through them), cataract surgery, surgery to fix the eye muscles, or Botox injections.

Figure 4: Faulty optics: When your vision isn't perfect

When the eye sees normally, light focuses directly on the retina, producing a clear image. But in some people, images appear blurred because the eye focuses light rays either in front of or behind the retina. These problems are not eye diseases, but common conditions known as refractive errors of the eye. Although laser surgery procedures such as LASIK have become increasingly popular as a way to correct refractive errors, these techniques are usually most appropriate for people younger than 50. For that reason, refractive errors in older adults are most often corrected with eyeglasses or contact lenses.

Myopia (nearsightedness). A nearsighted person has difficulty seeing objects at a distance because the light rays converge and focus before reaching the retina. The cause is usually an elongated eyeball (which requires light rays to travel farther than they would in a normal eye) or a lens or cornea that is too strong (which bends the light rays so much that they focus before reaching the retina).

Hyperopia (farsightedness). A farsighted person sees objects better at a distance than up close. In this case, the eyeball is usually too short, and light rays reach the retina before they are focused. Hyperopia can also be caused by weaknesses in the refractive power of the lens and cornea. You may not notice farsightedness for years, but because your eye's corrective ability diminishes with age, you will probably need glasses by midlife.

Astigmatism. A person with astigmatism has irregularities in the curvature of the cornea's surface that cause distorted vision. Light rays do not meet at a single point. For some people, vertical lines appear blurry; for others, horizontal or diagonal lines look out of focus. Astigmatism develops early and is usually well established after the first few years of life. It often occurs together with nearsightedness or farsightedness.

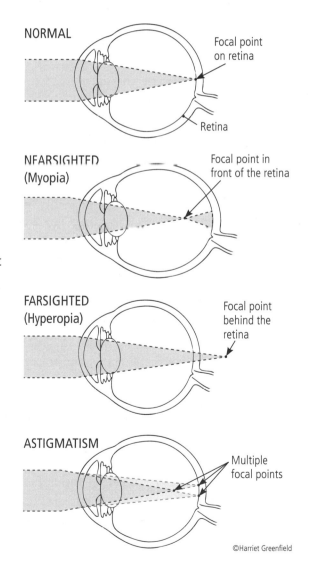

NORMAL — Focal point on retina — Retina

NEARSIGHTED (Myopia) — Focal point in front of the retina

FARSIGHTED (Hyperopia) — Focal point behind the retina

ASTIGMATISM — Multiple focal points

©Harriet Greenfield

Eyelid problems

Age, certain diseases, and some cosmetic treatments can affect the muscles and skin of the upper and lower eyelids. Often the problem affects your appearance and nothing more, but in other cases it may interfere with vision or cause eye irritation.

Blepharitis. Blepharitis is inflammation of the eyelids. It can be caused by a problem with the oil glands near the base of the eyelids, a bacterial infection, or skin conditions like rosacea or seborrheic dermatitis (dandruff of the scalp and eyebrows). Though blepharitis usually doesn't affect your sight, it can make your eyelids red, itchy, and swollen and leave your eyes red and watery. Your ophthalmologist might recommend treatments like artificial tears or a short course of steroid eye drops to relieve discomfort from blepharitis. You'll also get treated for the cause of the problem, for example, with anti-dandruff shampoo or antibiotics. It also helps to regularly clean your eyelids with a warm washcloth.

Ptosis. Over time, the upper eyelids may start to sag as the muscles that support them lose their strength. Eye injury, nervous system problems, and disease (such as diabetes or myasthenia gravis) can also cause this condition. Botox injections to eliminate wrinkles in the brow and forehead may also cause drooping, which can last as long as three months.

Although upper eyelid drooping is often only a cosmetic concern, it can interfere with sight if the lid is so lax that it covers or partially covers the pupil. Before trying any treatment, you will need a medical exam to identify the cause. If a disease caused your ptosis, the drooping usually improves when the disease is treated. If the problem is caused by Botox injections, it should resolve in about three to four months when the injection wears off.

If a droopy eyelid is unattractive or interferes with your vision and is not caused by a treatable disease, you may want to consider surgical repair. The ptosis repair procedure removes excess tissue and lifts the lid. It can be performed under local or general anesthesia on an outpatient basis. Many health insurers will cover this operation, but only if the ptosis affects your vision. Your ophthalmologist or oculoplastic specialist can determine whether you qualify for coverage.

Blepharochalasis. When eyelid skin loses elasticity and sags, it creates new folds that can droop over the lashes and block the upper field of sight by covering the pupil. In blepharochalasis, just the skin of the lid begins to droop, not the entire lid as in ptosis (which is caused by muscle weakening). A surgical procedure called blepharoplasty can correct this condition. As with ptosis, most health insurers will pay for this repair only if the condition interferes with vision.

Ectropion. This condition occurs when the muscles of the lower lid weaken, making the lid sag and turn outward, away from the eyeball. As a result, the upper and lower lids no longer meet when the eye is closed, and the eye may tear excessively. The constantly exposed cornea and conjunctiva may become red and irritated. In mild cases, no treatment is needed. You can use over-the-counter artificial tears and a plastic eye shield at night to hold moisture in your eye. If the symptoms or appearance bother you, surgery can tighten the lower eyelid and surrounding muscles. After the surgery, you may need to wear an eye patch for a few hours and apply antibiotic ointment for a few days.

Entropion. In this condition the lower lid rolls inward toward the eye. Because the lashes constantly rub against the cornea, entropion may produce irritation, a feeling of something in the eye, tearing, and blurring. In mild cases, it can help to tape the lower lid to the cheek every night so the edge of the lid and the lashes are in the proper position. Ask your doctor if this approach might work for you and find out how to do it properly. A surgeon can also correct this disorder with a relatively simple procedure that removes a piece of your lower eyelid to tighten the skin and muscles there.

Skin cancer. The eyelids are among the most common areas of the body for non-melanoma skin cancers like basal cell and squamous cell carcinomas. When you do a full-body mole check once a month or so, also examine your eyelids for any unusual growths that have changed color or shape. Alert your ophthalmologist if you notice anything unusual. Your doctor can examine the growth and decide whether it should be biopsied. If it is cancerous, an oculoplastic specialist will remove it and reconstruct the eyelid as necessary.

Dry eye syndrome

As people age, their tear production declines, producing irritation, burning, or a slightly painful, scratchy feeling in the eye. Sometimes mucus accumulates, causing a sticky sensation. You may become sensitive to light, have trouble wearing contact lenses, or even find it difficult to cry. When the problem is severe, it may feel like you have sand in your eyes. This combination of symptoms is called dry eye syndrome. Dry eye can also cause fluctuations in vision or blurred vision.

More than 16 million adults in the United States —11 million women and five million men—have dry eye syndrome. The likelihood of developing this condition increases as you age. Just under 3% of people ages 18 to 34 have dry eye syndrome. By age 75, about 19% of people are affected.

Dry eye is more common in people who have
- allergies
- blepharitis (inflammation of the eyelid)
- lupus or rheumatoid arthritis
- Parkinson's disease (which reduces blinking)
- Sjögren's syndrome (an immune system disorder)
- skin disorders like rosacea or seborrheic dermatitis.

Dry eye syndrome is also more common in people who take certain medications, such as antihistamines, decongestants, antidepressants, anticholinergics, and diuretics.

An ophthalmologist can diagnose dry eye syndrome with a slit lamp and can test the amount of tear production. A newer diagnostic test, TearLab, takes a small sample of tears to measure their osmolarity—

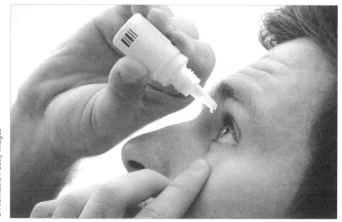

The simplest remedy for dry eye is eye drops. Others include special contact lenses to retain moisture and tiny plugs to block tear drainage.

▶ Symptoms of dry eye syndrome
- ✔ Persistent sensation of grittiness in the eyes
- ✔ Difficulty wearing contact lenses
- ✔ Inability to shed tears
- ✔ Burning sensation in low humidity or polluted air
- ✔ Fluctuations in vision
- ✔ Blurred vision that clears when you blink or use artificial tears

that is, their saltiness. When you have fewer tears, the ones that remain are saltier, and are therefore less healthy than usual.

If your dry eye is caused by a reduction in natural tear production, eye drops may help. For moderate to severe cases, treatment usually involves some type of topical medication (nonprescription artificial tears or ointments) or a prescription medication, such as topical cyclosporine (Restasis). Although dry eye may be sporadic, longtime sufferers often need to use these drugs regularly.

In 2016, the FDA approved the first in a new class of dry eye drugs, an eye drop called lifitegrast (Xiidra). Unlike Restasis, which increases tear production, Xiidra works by reducing inflammation in the eyes. Clinical studies found that Xiidra improved the symptoms of dry eye better than an inactive drop (placebo).

For more severe dry eye, doctors sometimes prescribe tears made from your own serum, the clear liquid part of your blood. The blood serum is diluted into a bottle of preserved artificial tears. Your doctor might also prescribe an eye insert such as hydroxypropyl cellulose (Lacrisert), which is placed between your lower eyelid and eyeball. As the insert dissolves, it slowly releases the same substance found in artificial tear eye drops to keep your eyes moist.

There's also a new, drug-free way to treat dry eye. TrueTear, which the FDA approved in 2017, is a handheld device that uses small pulses of energy to temporarily stimulate tear production. TrueTear has been shown to significantly increase tear production, but because you place the device in your nose, it can cause side effects like nasal pain, nosebleeds, and sneezing.

In severe cases of dry eye, an ophthalmologist may

recommend the insertion of temporary or permanent punctal plugs into the tear drainage ducts. These plugs prevent your natural tears from draining out of the opening in the inner corner of the eyelid. Alternatively, your doctor may prescribe special soft contact lenses that help hold in moisture. You may also be advised to wear goggles at night to retain moisture, especially if your eye does not fully close while you sleep.

To minimize evaporation of tears, avoid exposure to dust, pollen, cigarette smoke, and other pollutants. Also, stay out of the wind and away from hair dryers and air conditioner currents. Turn on a humidifier to add moisture to dry indoor air. Try to remember to blink frequently and fully, especially when you are reading or at the computer.

What you eat may also help keep your eyes moist. One study found that women who ate plenty of omega-3 fatty acids (a healthy fat found in tuna, salmon, and other fatty fish, as well as in flaxseed) were less likely to develop dry eye syndrome than women who rarely ate such fats. Tuna in particular seemed to be the most beneficial. However, taking omega-3s in supplement form may not help as much as previously thought, when it comes to treating dry eye. A study published in *The New England Journal of Medicine* in 2018 found that a 3,000-mg daily omega-3 supplement didn't significantly improve dry eye symptoms compared with a placebo dose of olive oil.

Another way to combat dry eye, as well as eye-strain, is to break the habit of staring at your computer

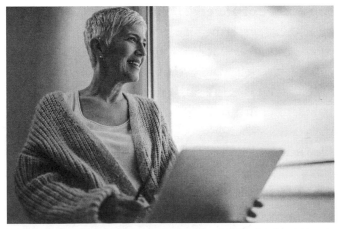

If you have dry eye, remember to blink frequently and fully, especially at the computer. Every 20 minutes, take a 20-second break to look away from your monitor. Then close your eyes for 20 seconds.

screen for hours at a time. Follow the 20-20-20-20 rule: Every 20 minutes, take a 20-second break and look away from your monitor. Focus on something that's at least 20 feet away. Then close your eyes for 20 seconds more.

Watery eyes

Although some people develop dry eyes as they grow older, others have the opposite problem—watery eyes. This may seem counterintuitive, but the problem often develops because of dry eye syndrome. Dry eyes are uncomfortable, which causes the eyes to reflexively produce more tears.

Watery eyes also can result from tear drainage problems. Normally tears drain from the surface of your eyes, flow under your eyelids, and pass down into the nasal passages. But if this drainage system gets blocked, tears can build up in the eyes until they spill over the lids. An eyelid problem or infection also can lead to watery eyes.

Your doctor may analyze a sample of your tears to see if an infection is to blame, or test your tear production. Another test involves irrigating the tear drainage system to check for possible blockages.

Treatment for watery eyes depends on the cause. If dry eye syndrome is causing excessive tearing, the treatment is the same as for dry eyes (see previous section). When an infection is responsible, your doctor will most likely prescribe antibiotics. Surgery can repair any blockage in the drainage system.

Corneal edema

The cornea—the clear, dome-shaped structure at the front of the eye—is essential to sharp vision. A layer of endothelial cells along the inner corneal surface keeps the cornea clear and compact by pumping fluid from the cornea into the aqueous humor. Any damage to or loss of these endothelial cells can cause fluid to build up in the cornea and vision to become cloudy.

You can lose these protective cells as a result of a disorder called Fuchs' dystrophy or after any surgery involving the inside of the eye (such as cataract, glaucoma, or retinal surgery). Both of these situations become more likely as you age. If you develop corneal edema, you may notice blurred vision or haloes—especially when you first wake up in the morning.

Mild corneal edema that doesn't interfere with your vision may not need to be treated. Your eye doctor might prescribe concentrated saline eye drops or ointment (sold as Muro 128) to pull the extra fluid out of your cornea.

Doctors have traditionally treated more severe, vision-obscuring corneal edema with a corneal transplant. A less invasive alternative to a total corneal transplant, called Descemet stripping endothelial keratoplasty (DSEK), involves removing just a small layer of diseased cells lining the cornea and replacing them with a graft of endothelial cells from a human donor. The graft is temporarily kept in place by an air bubble until it adheres.

Conjunctivitis

Conjunctivitis, also known as "pink eye," doesn't only affect children. This inflammation or infection of the conjunctiva—the clear layer lining the inner surface of the eyelid and the white of the eye—can occur at any age.

Signs that you might have conjunctivitis include
- itching or burning in the eyes
- discharge from one or both eyes
- a pinkish color to the whites of the eyes
- tearing and greater light sensitivity.

Four different types of conjunctivitis exist, and each type is treated slightly differently:

Allergic conjunctivitis is caused by an allergy to an airborne substance (such as seasonal pollen) or a foreign body in the eye (such as a contact lens). The best way to prevent it is to avoid the offending substance. You can treat mild cases with artificial tears.

More severe allergic conjunctivitis can be relieved with antihistamines, NSAIDs, or steroid eye drops.

Chemical conjunctivitis occurs after you've been exposed to an irritant, such as air pollution or chlorine in a swimming pool. You can treat it by flushing the eye with a saltwater solution (saline), then applying steroid drops.

Viral conjunctivitis is caused by the same types of viruses responsible for upper respiratory infections like the common cold. It should go away once the illness runs its course. To increase your comfort in the meantime, try artificial tears and cool compresses. Handwashing is very important, as viral conjunctivitis is highly contagious.

Bacterial conjunctivitis occurs from an infection with staphylococcal, streptococcal, or other bacteria, and it is contagious. This type of conjunctivitis is typically treated with antibiotic drops or ointment, but before your doctor prescribes an antibiotic, he or she may want to make sure that you actually have a bacterial infection. (A lab test of discharge from the affected eye can confirm the diagnosis.) A study in the journal *Ophthalmology* found that about 60% of people with conjunctivitis receive a prescription for antibiotic eye drops, even though most cases are caused by a virus and resolve on their own without medication.

Floaters

Older people often notice occasional spots or opaque flecks drifting across their line of vision, particularly when they look at a page of a book, a computer screen, or a solid, light background. These symptoms may be most noticeable when you are tired. Floaters are tiny clusters of cells or gel in the vitreous cavity, where the clear, jelly-like substance called vitreous humor fills your eyeball. What you actually see is the shadow these little clumps cast on the retina. In some cases, the vitreous gel may detach from the retina and suddenly cause more floaters—a condition known as posterior vitreous detachment.

About 25% of people have vitreous detachments and floaters by their 60s, and 65% have them by their 80s. Floaters also appear more often in people who are nearsighted, have had cataract surgery, or had a recent injury to their head or eyes. These phenomena are usually nothing more than an annoyance and often dissipate or become less bothersome on their own. However, if they occur suddenly or noticeably increase, consult an ophthalmologist. Certain eye diseases or injuries can cause floaters. Occasionally, floaters can be small drops of blood from a torn retinal vessel. Less commonly, new floaters are the sign of a retinal tear (See "Retinal tear or detachment," below).

Once floaters have been checked and declared harmless, one of three things may happen. A floater may disappear as it breaks apart or settles; it may become less noticeable with time as your brain pays less attention to it; or it may persist to the point where it becomes bothersome. Floaters can be removed, but the risk of surgery is often greater than the benefit of removing the floater. If floaters interfere with your central vision, moving the eye up and down or left and right may shift them out of your line of sight and provide temporary relief.

Flashes

Seeing shooting stars—a phenomenon called photopsia—is relatively common as people age. Solitary flashes appear as sparks or minuscule strands of light, almost like streaks of lightning across the sky. They occur when the vitreous gel bumps, rubs, or tugs against the retina. Flashes are generally harmless and require no treatment, but in rare cases, they may warn of more severe retinal complications (see "Retinal tear or detachment," below). If their appearance is sudden or accompanied by a shower of floaters or a loss of peripheral vision, call your ophthalmologist right away. Photopsia differs from the flashing or zigzag lights that may precede migraine headaches.

Retinal tear or detachment

Occasionally, floaters and flashes can be a sign of something far more serious: a retinal tear or retinal detachment. In a retinal tear, the vitreous gel pulls on the retina with enough force to tear the retina. Fluid from inside the eye may enter through this tear and separate the retina from the underlying tissues that nourish it. Separation of the retina from the back of the eye is called a retinal detachment.

People who are middle-aged and older are most likely to experience retinal detachment. Nearsightedness increases the chances for detachment, as do cataract removal surgery and eye injuries.

Retinal detachment is a serious condition that can lead to permanent vision loss. If you suspect that your retina is detaching, contact your ophthalmologist immediately. If you cannot reach your own doctor, go to an emergency room for evaluation. When a retinal tear is caught early, treatment may prevent detachment. Left untreated, the condition may worsen until the retina separates completely from the inner wall of the eye, remaining connected only at the optic nerve in the back of the eye and the ciliary body in the front of the eye. In the worst cases, retinal detachment causes blindness.

Because the underlying disorder that causes retinal tears may occur in both eyes, your ophthalmologist will want to examine both eyes thoroughly. Your other eye may also have retinal deterioration or other problems that require treatment.

A dilated eye exam using an indirect ophthalmoscope (a device that is mounted on special headgear) enables the doctor to determine the extent of the detachment and the location of any holes or tears. This can help the doctor determine the best way to treat the problem. Some retinal tears don't require treatment, especially if they are old. But most cases of retinal detachment call for surgery to reposition the separated retina against the back wall of the eye.

▶ Symptoms of retinal detachment

Contact your ophthalmologist immediately or go to the emergency department of your local hospital if you notice any of these early warning symptoms of retinal detachment:

✔ Flashing lights

✔ New or increased floaters

✔ Gradual shading of vision from one side (like a curtain being drawn)

✔ Rapid deterioration of sharp, central vision (this occurs when the macula detaches)

Doctors can choose among several surgical options.

Laser photocoagulation. In this procedure, which is done on an outpatient basis with topical anesthesia, the doctor uses pinpoints of laser light to create tiny burns around any small holes or tears in the retina. The resulting scar tissue forms a barrier that essentially welds the retina to the back wall of the eye so that it is less likely to detach (see Figure 5, at right).

Cryopexy. An ophthalmologist can repair tears that have not yet caused detachment by applying a freezing treatment called cryopexy. Like laser photocoagulation, this approach functions as spot welding for the retina, reducing the likelihood of the tear leading to a detachment. This procedure is performed on an outpatient basis using local anesthesia. It may be used when the location of a tear makes laser surgery too difficult to perform.

Pneumatic retinopexy. This approach is frequently used as the initial treatment for repairing a detached retina, because it can be done on an outpatient basis and it leads to the quickest vision recovery. Whether or not it will work for you depends on the location of your retinal tear (or tears) and the characteristics of the retinal detachment.

For this procedure, you receive local anesthesia to numb the eye. The ophthalmologist first uses cryopexy (or, less frequently, laser photocoagulation) to create a barrier with scar tissue. Then a gas bubble is injected into the vitreous cavity. As the gas bubble expands over the next few days, you are positioned in a way that allows the gas to hold the retina in place, enabling the cryopexy to seal off any holes and reattach the retina. Eventually the gas bubble dissipates, and fluid in the eye takes its place.

The most challenging aspect of this procedure may be the recovery. To ensure that the retina reattaches properly, you may have to spend a significant amount of time each day in a face-down position to keep the bubble in the correct place. Until the gas bubble disappears, you should also arrange pillows in your bed to

Figure 5: Laser photocoagulation

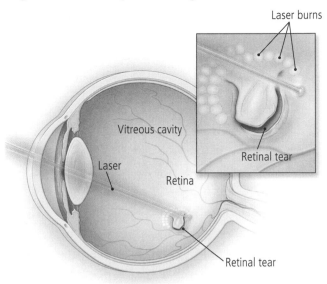

In this procedure, which is usually done in an office, the ophthalmologist uses a laser to make a series of tiny burns around the retinal tear. This creates a barrier of scar tissue that stops the tear from getting worse.

prevent you from lying on your back. Your eye doctor can provide more specific advice.

Scleral buckling. This procedure, which is done in an operating room while you are under local or general anesthesia, drains the fluid so the retina falls back against the choroid. The hole is sealed, and then a silicone buckle is sutured around the outside of the eyeball to slightly indent the sclera (the white outer layer of the eyeball) so that it makes better contact with the retina. In addition to this procedure, you will undergo cryopexy or laser therapy, and a gas bubble may be injected to keep the retina in place.

Vitrectomy. This surgery is usually performed under local anesthesia. The surgeon removes the vitreous humor that might be causing traction or tugging on the retina, and performs cryopexy or laser treatment. Then the vitreous humor is replaced with a saline solution or a gas bubble that dissipates and is gradually replaced with fluid that the eye makes on its own. ◗

Safeguarding your sight

Although aging puts people at greater risk for serious eye diseases, vision loss does not have to go hand in hand with growing old. Practical, preventive measures can help protect against devastating eye changes. Importantly, an estimated 40% to 50% of all blindness can be avoided or treated with proper care.

Eye exams are the cornerstone of visual health as you age. Anyone with a family history of eye disease or other risk factors should have more frequent exams. (For guidelines on how often to be examined, see Table 1, page 17.) *Don't wait until your vision deteriorates to have an eye exam.* One eye can often compensate for the other, while an eye condition develops or progresses without your knowledge. Frequently, only an exam can detect eye disease in its earliest stages, when it is most treatable.

Beyond regular eye exams, there are also practical steps that everyone should take to help prevent damage to the eyes. These include adapting your lifestyle and protecting your eyes from dangerous exposures.

The eye examination

Regular, comprehensive eye exams are the best way to detect eye disease early, when treatment is most effective. A thorough eye exam involves a series of evaluations—some done in the dark, some in the light, and some with special instruments. People with sensitive eyes or a fear of eye exams should be assured that the experience is not painful.

Because some eye disorders are inherited and others develop after an illness, the doctor will ask about your family and personal health history. Diabetes, for example, can affect vision and always deserves careful attention (see "Diabetic retinopathy," page 47).

In addition to the tests described here, others may be performed if you have a specific eye condition, such as glaucoma.

Testing your vision

The familiar set of rows of letters and numbers that diminish in size is called the Snellen chart. A doctor or technician uses this chart to test the sharpness of your central vision, known as visual acuity. Think of central vision as your eye's most important vital sign, much like blood pressure and heart rate are your heart's essential

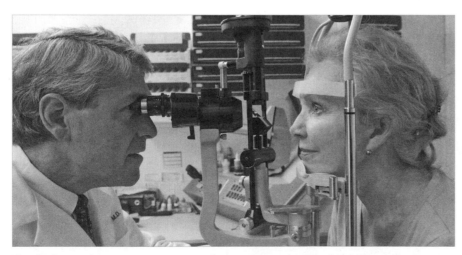

The single most important step you can take to protect your vision is having regular eye exams. These can enable you to detect and treat problems early.

© Huntstock | Getty Images

Table 1: How often do you need routine eye exams?

OTHERWISE HEALTHY PEOPLE WITH NO RISK FACTORS	
Younger than 40	Get a vision screening once every three years, but see an ophthalmologist if you are having problems
Ages 40 to 64	Get a complete eye exam from an ophthalmologist once every two to four years to monitor for glaucoma and a vision screening to correct for presbyopia
Ages 65 and older	Get a complete eye exam every one to two years
PEOPLE AT HIGH RISK FOR EYE DISEASES	
Type 1 diabetes	Get a complete eye exam five years after diagnosis, then once a year
Type 2 diabetes	Get a complete eye exam at the time of diagnosis, then once a year
At risk for glaucoma, ages 40 to 54	Get a complete eye exam every one to three years
At risk for glaucoma, ages 55 to 64	Get a complete eye exam every one to two years
At risk for glaucoma, ages 65 or older	Get a complete eye exam every six to 12 months
PEOPLE WHO ALREADY HAVE AN EYE DISEASE	

- You may need more frequent eye examinations. Ask your ophthalmologist what's right for you.

- You may also need more frequent exams if you are taking certain medications, such as amiodarone (Cordarone), ethambutol (Myambutol), hydroxychloroquine (Plaquenil), prednisone, or tamoxifen (Nolvadex). Ask your doctor for guidance.

vital signs. If you wear corrective lenses, the doctor will test your vision while you wear your glasses or contact lenses and will also look at your glasses through a device called a lensometer to determine their prescription.

Your exam score indicates how well you see compared with someone whose vision is normal. For instance, if you have 20/20 vision—considered the standard for normal—you can see at a distance of 20 feet what another individual with normal vision sees at 20 feet. However, if your vision is 20/40, you see at a distance of 20 feet what a person with normal vision would be able to see at 40 feet; in other words, you need to stand closer to the object to see it as clearly. In general, the higher the second number, the worse your vision.

If the test indicates that you need corrective lenses or a prescription adjustment, your doctor will measure your eye's refraction, or focusing accuracy, using instruments that contain a combination of corrective lenses. To confirm that reading, you will be asked to look through a variety of lenses to ascertain which one gives you the best sight. The numbers in your eyeglass prescription indicate the amount of lens power correction you need for nearsightedness (marked by a minus sign) or farsightedness (marked by a plus sign). For example, -9 is highly nearsighted, while -1 is mildly nearsighted.

The doctor examines the pupils to make sure they are reacting normally to light. The next step is generally an evaluation of your peripheral vision. Typically you'll be asked to cover one eye and focus the other eye on a point straight ahead. The doctor may shift an object, such as a pen, back and forth at the outer edges of your visual field and ask you to note when you see it moving.

In certain circumstances, your color vision may also be measured with special color pictures. In addition, the doctor can test your depth perception with a series of three-dimensional images. This is especially important if anyone in your family has had strabismus (eye muscle imbalance).

Examining the external eye

Assessing the coordination of the six muscles in each eye is an important part of the exam, to ensure that your eyes function properly together. The doctor will ask you to look straight up, to the right, and so forth.

The doctor might also check the positioning of your eyelids to make sure they aren't drooping, and evaluate your blink reflex. In addition, the external eye examination includes a check of your eyeball's outer structures (including the cornea, iris, sclera, and conjunctiva).

Using a slit lamp—a diagnostic tool with a powerful microscope and a narrow slit of light—the doctor can explore both the external and internal parts of your eyes. When examining the outer part of the eye, the doctor uses the slit lamp to check your lids, lashes, and orbit and to look for any signs of underlying problems, such as infections, sties, cysts, tumors, or lid muscle weakness.

Examining the internal eye

The slit lamp's narrow light beam and high magnification provide a cross-sectional picture of the eye's inner structures as well. This gives the doctor a close-up view of the anterior chamber, lens, vitreous humor, and retina. The doctor will check for many things, including inflammation in the anterior chamber and clouding of the lens (cataracts).

Testing with pupil dilation. The doctor applies special eye drops to dilate your pupils so he or she can thoroughly examine the retina. The drops take time to wear off, so people often experience light sensitivity and difficulty focusing on close tasks for several hours afterward. Be aware that it is often difficult to drive while your eyes are dilated. You may want to have someone drive you home.

Measuring eye pressure (tonometry). This painless test for eye pressure can detect signs of glaucoma and is also used to monitor glaucoma treatment. The simplest version, known as air-puff or non-contact tonometry, uses an instrument called a tonometer that emits a puff of air to determine what force it takes to flatten the cornea. Anyone at risk for glaucoma, including those who are over age 40 or who have a borderline result on the air-puff test, should be given a more accurate test, known as applanation tonometry. After the eye is numbed with anesthetic drops, the doctor gently touches the cornea with an instrument to measure the eye's internal pressure.

Viewing the retina and optic nerve. Finally, the doctor will use a hand-held ophthalmoscope or focusing lenses with a light source (mounted on the doctor's head

Your eye professionals

If you've ever been confused about whether you need to see an ophthalmologist, optometrist, or optician, you're not alone. Although the names of these specialists sound similar, each plays a distinct role in eye care. Because the training and experience of each specialist varies, it is important to seek the services of the appropriate professional for your eye care needs.

Ophthalmologist. An ophthalmologist is a physician—either a doctor of medicine (M.D.) or a doctor of osteopathy (D.O.)—who specializes in the medical and surgical care of the eyes and visual system, as well as in the prevention of eye disease. Licensed ophthalmologists must complete four or more years of medical school, one year of internship, and three or more years of specialized medical, surgical, and refractive training. Ophthalmologists are qualified to diagnose and treat (medically and surgically) diseases, disorders, and injuries of the eyes and visual system. In addition, they can provide more basic eye care, including prescribing eyeglasses and contact lenses.

Oculoplastic specialist. This is an ophthalmologist who has received advanced training in plastic and reconstructive surgery of the eye and surrounding structures. Oculoplastic specialists are often consulted for problems with the eyelids, tear drainage, and skin cancer around the eyes.

Optometrist. An optometrist, or doctor of optometry, is a health service provider who evaluates and treats vision problems. Optometrists must complete a four-year course at an accredited college of optometry, but they do not attend medical school and are not trained to perform surgery. They are licensed by their state to examine the eyes, determine the presence of vision problems (including eye diseases), and prescribe eyeglasses and contact lenses. In many states, optometrists are permitted to treat certain eye conditions with medications. Normally, if an optometrist diagnoses a serious eye disorder in a patient, he or she will refer that person to an ophthalmologist.

Optician. An optician is a technician who makes and fits eyeglasses, contact lenses, or other optical devices that have been prescribed by an ophthalmologist or optometrist.

Investing in the right sunglasses

The easiest way to protect your eyes from the sun's hazardous radiation is to wear sunglasses, not only in the summer months, but year-round. Ultraviolet (UV) light can damage the iris, retina, lens, and cornea, leading to permanent vision loss. It's a good idea to request UV protection (an invisible coating) on all of your prescription glasses.

UV light has three wavelengths:

UVA is long, looks almost blue in the visible spectrum, and is responsible for skin tanning and aging.

UVB is shorter and more energetic, and it's linked to sunburn and skin cancer. A large portion of UVB light is absorbed by the atmosphere's ozone layer.

UVC is short. It is completely absorbed by the ozone layer.

Sunglasses are labeled according to guidelines for UV protection established by the American National Standards Institute (ANSI). There are three categories:

Cosmetic. These lightly tinted lenses are good for daily wear. They block 70% of UVB rays, 20% of UVA, and 60% of visible light.

General purpose. These medium to dark lenses are fine for most outdoor recreation. They block 95% of UVB, 60% of UVA, and 60% to 90% of visible light. Most sunglasses fall into this category.

Special purpose. These are extremely dark lenses with UV blockers, recommended for places with very bright conditions, such as beaches and ski slopes. They block 99% of UVB, 60% of UVA, and 97% of visible light.

Just because a lens is expensive or appears darker doesn't mean that its ability to block out UV radiation is any greater than that of a cheaper or

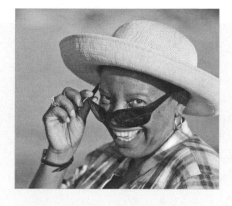

lighter lens. Look for the ANSI label. Even inexpensive sunglasses can be protective.

There is some evidence that blue light from the sun may contribute to the development of age-related macular degeneration. Lenses with a red, amber, or orange tint may provide better protection against this light. You may find less distortion, however, with gray or green lenses.

If you aren't sure what kind of sunglasses to buy or think you may be at high risk for eye disease, ask an eye care professional for a recommendation.

---

or on the slit lamp) to look more deeply into your eye. This exam evaluates the clarity of the lens and vitreous humor, and the health of the retina, macula, optic nerve, and their blood vessels. In special circumstances, the doctor will use different lenses to view the far periphery of the retina.

Practical steps

You can take other steps on your own to protect and preserve your vision. Following are some of the most important things you can do.

Don't smoke. The chemicals in cigarette smoke travel through the network of tiny blood vessels that supply your macula. Eventually, those chemicals can damage the blood vessels and lead to age-related macular degeneration. Smoking has also been linked to an increased risk for cataracts, in part by increasing the production of damaging molecules called free radicals in the lens and reducing the amount of protective antioxidants that help disarm the free radicals. In addition, people who smoke are more likely to develop uveitis (eye inflammation) and diabetic retinopathy, and to have more severe cases of dry eye.

Wear sunglasses and a hat. The right protective gear will shield your eyes from the damaging effects of ultraviolet (UV) radiation, which has been linked to conditions like cataracts and age-related macular degeneration. For tips on choosing sunglasses, see "Investing in the right sunglasses," above. Your hat should have at least a three-inch brim.

Eat a balanced nutritious diet, with plenty of fruits and vegetables. Just as sunglasses and a hat protect your eyes from the outside, the right foods can protect your vision from the inside,

© RichLegg | Getty Images

helping to ward off certain eye diseases. For example, studies show that people who eat the most foods rich in the antioxidants lutein and zeaxanthin (such as spinach and other dark-green vegetables) are less likely to develop cataracts and age-related macular degeneration.

These nutrients filter out harmful blue wavelengths of light, protecting your eye cells from damage. It's also a good idea to minimize saturated fats and hydrogenated oils, which contribute to blood vessel damage and can diminish blood flow to your eyes.

Common eye myths dispelled

Myth: Doing eye exercises will delay the need for glasses.

Fact: Eye exercises will not improve or preserve vision or reduce the need for glasses. Your vision depends on many factors, including the shape of your eye and the health of the eye tissues, none of which can be significantly altered with eye exercises.

Myth: Reading in dim light will worsen your vision.

Fact: Dim lighting is unlikely to adversely affect your eyesight. However, it will tire your eyes out more quickly. The best way to position a reading light is as close to your book, newspaper, or magazine as possible, so that it shines directly onto the page. If possible, use a desk lamp with an opaque shade and point it directly at the reading material.

Myth: Carrots are the best food for the eyes.

Fact: Carrots, which contain vitamin A, are indeed good for the eyes. But fresh fruits and dark-green leafy vegetables, which contain more antioxidant vitamins such as C and E, are even better. Antioxidant vitamins may help protect the eyes against cataracts and age-related macular degeneration. Just don't expect them to prevent or correct basic vision problems such as nearsightedness or farsightedness.

Myth: It's best not to wear glasses all the time. Taking a break from glasses or contact lenses allows your eyes to rest.

Fact: If you need glasses for distance or reading, use them. Attempting to read without reading glasses will simply strain your eyes and tire them out. Using your glasses won't worsen your vision or lead to eye disease.

Myth: Staring at a computer screen all day is bad for the eyes.

Fact: Using a computer will not damage your eyes. However, staring at a computer screen all day will contribute to eyestrain or tired eyes. Adjust lighting so that it does not create a glare or harsh reflection on the screen. When you work on a computer or do other close work such as reading or sewing, it's a good idea to look away every 20 minutes for 20 seconds to lessen eye fatigue. People who stare at a computer screen for long periods tend not to blink as often as usual, which dries out the eyes. Make a conscious effort to blink regularly to keep your eyes well lubricated.

Wear safety glasses or goggles. An estimated 2.4 million eye injuries occur in the United States each year, and 90% of them would have been preventable with the use of appropriate safety eyewear. Put on protective goggles or safety glasses whenever you work with power tools, use cleaning supplies or other chemicals, or play sports. If you do get chemicals in your eyes, immediately flush them with water in the sink or shower for 15 minutes. Do not bandage your eyes. Seek medical care immediately.

Limit your screen time. Spending many hours in front of a television or computer screen or working in poor light does not cause harmful medical conditions (see "Common eye myths dispelled," at left), but it can fatigue your eyes. Follow the 20-20-20-20 rule: for every 20 minutes you spend looking at your computer screen, look away at something at least 20 feet away for 20 seconds or more, and then close your eyes for 20 seconds to give them a rest.

Learn about your own eye risks. Know your personal risks for eye problems and take preventive steps; for instance, if you have diabetes, controlling your blood sugar can delay both the start and progression of retinopathy. You should be able to recognize the warning signs of vision problems, so you can see a doctor before a condition causes further damage. ◗

Cataracts

Nearly 26 million Americans over age 40 have cataracts, and that number is expected to increase to almost 46 million by the year 2050. A cataract is a clouding of the normally clear lens of the eye. The condition got its name because looking through a clouded lens is like looking through a cataract, or large waterfall.

It takes years for the lens to become foggy, but the opacity can eventually cause a disabling loss of vision, either by distorting light rays or keeping them from reaching the retina at all. While some people develop cataracts in their 40s and 50s, most cataracts that are significant enough to cause vision loss occur after age 60. The average age for cataract surgery in the United States is the early to mid-70s.

What causes cataracts?

Contrary to what some people believe, cataracts are not caused by a film blanketing the eye; nor are they related to overuse of the eyes. They do not spread from one eye to the other—although the condition can develop in both eyes.

Aging and accompanying changes in the protein composition of the lens are the most common causes. Many cataracts develop as part of a normal aging process known as sclerosis or hardening. The lens becomes less resilient, less transparent, and often thicker. Fibers in the lens compress, and the lens stiffens. Clarity fades as proteins clump together, creating tiny specks or wheel-like spokes in the outer edges of the lens. In later stages, the milkiness becomes denser and occurs in the center of vision, making it difficult to see (see Figure 6, below left). The change in the lens is similar to what happens when you cook an egg white—it goes from clear to opaque. Early on, before cataracts cloud vision, they can cause nearsightedness, double vision, or distorted vision.

Most cataracts result from age-related changes in the lens. But other factors, such as family history, eye injuries, the use of some medications (particularly corticosteroids such as prednisone), and certain health problems (such as diabetes) can also contribute (see "Are you at risk for cataracts?" on page 22). Several studies have linked cataracts with alcohol consumption and smoking. Even if you have smoked for many years, quitting now will help lower the chances of cataracts forming in the future. Long-term exposure to high levels of ultraviolet-B (UVB) rays from the sun is another hazard, and studies have found a greater prevalence of cataracts in people who live in areas with abundant sunlight. Wearing sunglasses can help protect your eyesight and minimize cataract formation.

Figure 6: Cataract vision

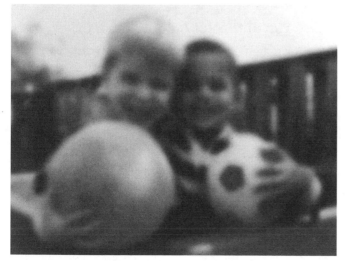

As cataracts progress, your vision gradually blurs or dims.

Photo courtesy of the National Eye Institute.

Diagnosing cataracts

Cataracts are painless and progress slowly. Vision usually turns blurry, hazy, or dim, and glare from lights and the sun can be bothersome. In the early stages, the eye may become more nearsighted because the denser the lens, the greater its refracting power. Night vision worsens, and colors appear duller. Because most cataracts develop very slowly, many people don't discover the problem until the loss of visual clarity forces them to make frequent changes to their eyeglass or contact lens prescriptions. These efforts eventually become fruitless, however, because corrective lenses don't help once the cataract becomes fairly dense.

Anyone who experiences blurry or dim vision should visit an ophthalmologist for a full examination. The doctor will test the sharpness of your vision with a traditional eye chart and may test how light scatters inside your eye (creating problems with glare). He or she will probably dilate your pupils with drops. By examining the interior of the eye with a slit lamp, the doctor can see the cataract and assess its severity. Additional tests will help rule out other eye disorders, such as glaucoma or retinal disease.

Preventing cataracts

There is no sure way to avoid developing cataracts. However, because of the link between cataracts and the sun's ultraviolet radiation, make sure to wear sunglasses as well as a hat or visor whenever you are outdoors (see "Investing in the right sunglasses," page 19). Smoking also appears to raise the risk of cataracts, so if you smoke, get advice from your doctor on how to quit.

Eating plenty of antioxidant-rich fruits and vegetables seems to make people less likely to develop cataracts. Especially helpful are spinach and other dark-green vegetables, which are rich in lutein and zeaxanthin. The AREDS2 study investigated whether high vitamin and mineral intake might reduce the risk for cataracts and advanced age-related macular degen-eration. Researchers found that people with very little lutein and zeaxanthin in their diet who took supplements of these nutrients lowered their risk of having cataract surgery by 32%.

Vitamin C might also be beneficial for stalling cataracts. A 2016 study of 324 female twin pairs, published in the journal *Ophthalmology*, found that participants with a diet rich in vitamin C had a 33% lower risk of cataract progression and clearer lenses after 10 years than those who ate less of this nutrient. The fluid that nourishes the lens and protects it from clouding is high in vitamin C. Making more of this nutrient available to the eye can have a protective effect, the authors say. They found that environmental factors including diet outweighed genes by roughly two to one when it came to explaining why cataracts progressed more quickly in some people.

Coping with early cataracts

In the early stages of cataract formation, you might notice a slight decline in your vision, but not so much that it affects your day-to-day activities. In some cases, the lens simply thickens, causing nearsightedness, rather than becoming opaque. In these instances, the following tips can help:

- Get a new eyeglass prescription if it improves your distance vision.
- Get antireflective coating on your lenses.

▶ Symptoms of cataracts

- ✔ Blurry or dim vision
- ✔ Glare from bright lights
- ✔ Double vision
- ✔ Faded colors
- ✔ Pale circles (called halos) around lights
- ✔ Declining night vision

Are you at risk for cataracts?

Age is the most common risk factor for cataracts. By age 80, more than half of Americans have developed a cataract. You are at higher risk for this common eye problem if you

- smoke
- use oral or inhaled corticosteroid medications (commonly prescribed for asthma, inflammatory bowel disease, rheumatoid arthritis, and other illnesses)
- have had an eye injury
- have diabetes
- have spent considerable time in the sun
- are obese
- are an alcoholic
- have a family history of cataracts.

Source: American Academy of Ophthalmology.

- Increase lighting at home, particularly for close work.
- Reduce glare by positioning lights as directly as possible on the task at hand, and by shielding your eyes from direct light.

These measures help many people successfully delay cataract surgery for years. Some end up never needing surgery.

Do you need cataract surgery?

Surgical removal of the clouded lens is the only effective cure for a cataract. No drugs, eye drops, diets, exercises, or glasses can reverse the problem. For most people, the only question is when to undergo the procedure. That decision is usually based on how much the cataract is interfering with vision.

The questionnaire "Should you consider cataract surgery?" (at right) can help you determine how much your vision loss is affecting your daily activities and when you should consider an operation. People who rely on their eyes for detailed work—such as architects, dentists, and jewelers—are likely to require surgery sooner than others. Driving is another consideration (see "Driving safely as you age," page 24). You should be able to delay cataract surgery until you feel that you need better vision, but timely cataract surgery can increase your safety when driving and lower your risk of falls.

Having cataract surgery might also extend your life, according to findings published in 2018 in *JAMA Ophthalmology*. In a 20-year study of more than 74,000 women enrolled in the Woman's Health Initiative, cataract surgery was associated with a 60% lower risk of death during the study period. Overall death rates dropped, as did rates of death from specific conditions like cancer, lung disease, and infections. The authors don't know the exact reason for the improved longevity, but their study provides another good incentive for moving forward with the procedure.

If your doctor determines that you have cataracts in both eyes, he or she may recommend operating first on the eye with the denser cataract (and poorer vision). If surgery is successful and your vision improves substantially, you may elect to forgo surgery

Should you consider cataract surgery?

If you answer "yes" to more than a few of these questions, consider having a consultation with an ophthalmologist.

Even with glasses, do you have difficulty
- reading a newspaper or book?
- seeing steps or curbs?
- reading traffic signs, street signs, or store signs?
- taking part in sports such as bowling, handball, tennis, or golf?
- watching television?
- seeing well in poor or dim light?
- recognizing people, even when they're close to you?

Do you experience
- glare caused by bright lights or street lights?
- blurry or hazy vision?
- halos or rings around lights?
- poor color vision?

Do you
- avoid driving because of your vision?
- have difficulty driving at night?

on your other eye. However, most people note significant benefits from having the second eye operation, including better depth perception and improvements in their ability to drive and to read.

Many people choose to have the second surgery once the first eye has healed and vision is stable. If you are extremely farsighted or nearsighted and need cataract surgery in both eyes, you may want to have the second surgery within about one month of the first operation. Otherwise, you might have problems with double vision and depth perception because of the difference in the eyeglasses prescription between your eyes. These problems will generally resolve once you've had surgery in both eyes.

Some people with cataracts have an additional eye problem, such as age-related macular degeneration. In some cases, your doctor may recommend cataract surgery because the cataracts make it difficult to examine and manage the other problem. Whatever your situation, you and your doctor should discuss the rationale for the operation, as well as its benefits and risks.

Types of cataract surgery

Cataract surgery is the most common eye operation—and among the most common surgeries—in the United States, with 3.7 million of these procedures performed each year. Once an inpatient procedure requiring up to a week of hospitalization, cataract surgery today is performed under local anesthesia on an outpatient basis. It is considered one of the safest of all surgeries. Most ophthalmologists either are trained to perform cataract surgery or can refer you to someone who is. Ask around to find an experienced surgeon.

Cataract surgery involves removing the clouded natural lens and replacing it with an artificial substitute. There are a variety of approaches for doing this.

Traditional procedures

Unlike some other eye surgeries, traditional cataract surgery does not use lasers, except in some follow-up. (For laser-assisted surgery, see the next section, below right.) To remove the original lens, the surgeon makes a tiny incision in the eye, a delicate procedure done with the aid of special microsurgical instruments and a surgical microscope. The doctor may choose between two main procedures for extracting the lens: phacoemulsification and extracapsular surgery.

Phacoemulsification. This procedure requires only a tiny (2–3 mm) incision in the cornea that often needs no stitches and heals rapidly. Through this incision, the doctor inserts a thin probe that releases ultrasound waves. The waves break the clouded lens into tiny pieces. The doctor then suctions out the pieces. The outer lining of the lens capsule (the membrane that surrounds the lens) is left behind to support the artificial lens implant (see Figure 7, page 25). The new lens is folded and inserted through the same incision using a small tool. Phacoemulsification—informally known as phaco—offers good long-term results. More than 97% of cases performed by an experienced surgeon are successful and free from complications.

Extracapsular surgery. This older technique is now typically reserved for very dense or hard cataracts. The surgeon makes an incision about three-eighths of an inch wide (9–10 mm) in the sclera (the white of the eye) under the upper eyelid, above the spot where the sclera and cornea join. The surgeon then opens the lens capsule and removes the harder, central portion of the clouded lens manually, usually in one piece, and then gently vacuums out the softer part of the lens. The outer part of the lens capsule is left undisturbed, providing support for a replacement lens. After putting in the new lens, the surgeon stitches up the incision.

The main difference between extracapsular surgery and phacoemulsification is that with phaco, most people can resume their normal routine sooner because the smaller incision heals faster. Both procedures restore vision to 20/40 or better in more than 90% of cases.

Laser-assisted procedures

Surgeons typically remove clouded lenses by hand using a metal or diamond-edged blade. But new techniques allow surgeons to make incisions and break

▶ **Driving safely as you age**

Elderly drivers have one real advantage—experience. All those years behind the wheel are invaluable when it comes to making sound driving decisions. Yet the detrimental effects of aging on the eyes and other senses can make safe driving more difficult, especially if you have an eye condition such as cataracts, macular degeneration, presbyopia, or glaucoma. Stay safe by getting annual eye exams, checking in with your ophthalmologist, and taking necessary precautions.

Invest in new, more powerful glasses to compensate for vision loss. Consider adding antireflective coating to your eyeglasses to reduce the temporary blindness from oncoming headlights at night. Cataracts make night driving particularly difficult.

You can also adjust your car to suit your needs. Consider installing broader side-view and rear-view mirrors to provide greater peripheral vision, or choose a car with bigger and brighter gauges to accommodate for the loss of near vision. Also think about adjusting your driving routine. Avoid potentially dangerous situations, like driving in heavy rain or in poorly lit areas at night, especially if you have cataracts.

To improve your driving skills, take a senior driver safety course offered by the AARP (www.aarp.org/families/driver_safety) or AAA (https://seniordriving.aaa.com). These courses will teach you how to compensate for the loss of vision, hearing, cognitive function, and motor function, and anticipate potential driving-related side effects of any medications you take.

up a cataract with a femtosecond laser. The pieces are then suctioned out, as in phacoemulsification.

Femtosecond laser–assisted cataract surgery (FLACS) may provide certain advantages over traditional surgery, theoretically allowing a higher degree of safety, efficiency, and precision. For example, creating the corneal incision with a laser rather than with a blade could reduce the likelihood of complications, such as astigmatism or wound leakage. In addition, to reach the lens, the surgeon must first make a tiny (5 mm) circular opening in the front part of the clear capsule surrounding the lens. This step, called an anterior capsulotomy, is very delicate, because the remainder of the capsule can't be damaged—it must be kept intact to hold the new lens in place. Performing the capsulotomy with a laser may be more accurate than with a needle. However, all of these potential advantages to this newer technology have yet to be confirmed by studies.

On the negative side, FLACS is more expensive than traditional phacoemulsification, and it is not covered by Medicare or most private insurance plans—nor is it likely to be covered anytime soon. Experts say the added costs may not be worth the potential benefits. Also, laser-assisted cataract surgery is not yet available at every medical center.

Figure 7: Traditional cataract surgery (phacoemulsification)

1.

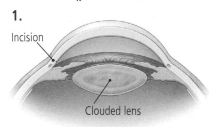

Incision

Clouded lens

The ophthalmologist makes a small incision about an eighth of an inch long in the side of the cornea.

2.

Phacoemulsifier

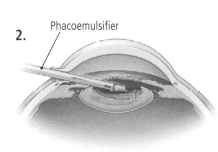

Using a small, needle-like probe called a phacoemulsifier, the doctor directs high-frequency sound waves through the lens to break it into small pieces, which are then gently suctioned out through the probe.

3.

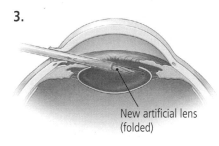

New artificial lens (folded)

The artificial lens, which is folded to fit inside a small inserter, is placed into the capsular bag through the same corneal incision.

4.

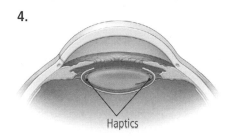

Haptics

The new lens unfolds inside the lens capsule and is held in place by tiny loops called haptics.

Replacement lenses

After your clouded lens is removed, a clear artificial lens called an intraocular lens (IOL) is implanted to replace it. Many factors affect your choice of IOL. Here are some questions your surgeon might ask:

- How do you feel about continuing to wear glasses or contact lenses after your cataract surgery?
- How important is good night vision for your lifestyle?
- In general, how well do you adjust to changes and learn new skills?
- What activities or tasks are part of your daily life, both for work and pleasure?
- During which activities would you find glasses the most inconvenient or aggravating?

There are several types of IOLs—monofocal, multifocal, accommodating, and toric—each with pluses and minuses. Some newer types of lenses address specific problems, such as reduced night vision.

Monofocal IOLs. Most people who have cataract surgery receive monofocal IOLs—lenses with a single focal length, like an ordinary pair of glasses. Monofocal lenses offer excellent contrast sensitivity and quality of vision, and they are covered by insurance. But they have limitations. These fixed-focus lenses can help you *either* see well without glasses at a distance (in which case you will need reading glasses to see up close) *or* see well without glasses for near work (in which case you will need glasses for distance activities like watching TV or driving). Some people who choose monofocal IOLs have one eye fitted with a lens that provides near vision and the other eye fitted with a lens that provides far vision. This combination, called monovision, is designed to decrease dependence on glasses. If you are considering this option, your eye surgeon may recommend that you try out monovision with contact lenses before your cataract surgery to see how well you adjust to this. Monovision is usually not an ideal option for people who require crisp, detailed vision or for those who have problems with depth perception or balance.

If you are going to receive monofocal IOLs and you also have astigmatism, you can have a procedure called astigmatic keratotomy at the same time as the cataract surgery. In this procedure, the surgeon makes small incisions in the cornea that help correct the shape of the eyeball, reducing the astigmatism.

Multifocal IOLs. Like bifocals or the progressive lenses used in glasses, these IOLs have different areas for distance, intermediate, and near vision. The brain and eye figure out which part of the lens to use. One example, the ReStor IOL, uses a type of refractive technology to provide focus at multiple distances. The lens has small, concentric circular ridges that permit the eye to change its range of focus. Another lens, called the ReZoom, has five broad zones to provide distance, intermediate, and near vision. Some newer multifocal IOLs also correct astigmatism. The main drawback of multifocal lenses is they can distort bright light, creating more glare and halos at night. Even though these lenses contain multiple focal lengths, you may still need glasses, and they are not covered by insurance.

Accommodating IOLs. These lenses do not have multiple focal lengths built in, but they can shift (or accommodate) from near to far vision in response to movements of the ciliary muscles in your eye, similar to the natural lens in a younger eye. These IOLs offer excellent distance and middle vision, but they aren't as reliable for near vision. Eye exercises can help you get used to accommodating lenses, but about half of peo-

ple who receive them end up needing reading glasses. Accommodating lenses are not covered by insurance.

Toric IOLs. These specialized monofocal IOLs are designed for people with a type of astigmatism known as regular astigmatism. One drawback to toric IOLs is the risk that they can rotate out of position, which may require further surgery to reposition or replace the lens. They are also not covered by insurance.

Newer lenses
IOLs have come a long way in the last few years. Companies that make these lenses are interested in enhancing quality of vision after cataract surgery, not just minimizing need for glasses.

Aspheric IOLs. Unlike traditional IOLs, which are spherical (meaning the front surface is uniformly curved), aspheric IOLs are slightly flatter around the edges. These lenses may improve your ability to distinguish an object from its background and reduce glare and halos.

Light-blocking IOLs. A few IOLs include filters that block blue light, the type of light that is thought to increase the risk of age-related macular degeneration and other vision problems. However, some experts say the protection these lenses provide is no better than that of the eye's natural lens, and that people who receive non-light-blocking IOLs can simply wear sunglasses in bright light to reduce their risk of developing these vision issues.

Three-piece light-adjustable lens. This experimental technology allows the surgeon to adjust the power of the lens by shining an ultraviolet light on it. As the light hits the lens, it changes shape to correct vision. The doctor can make adjustments several weeks after surgery, once the eye has healed and vision has become stable.

Preparing for cataract surgery
Before surgery, the doctor will measure the curvature of your cornea and the length of your eye to calculate the power of the implant you need. You'll also have a general medical exam to assess your overall health.

You may need to avoid certain drugs before surgery. For example, aspirin and other drugs with an anticoagulant (blood-thinning) effect can increase your risk of bleeding during surgery. (Cataract surgery is generally considered low risk for major bleeding complications.) If you can't stop taking blood thinners because you're at high risk for a blood clot, your eye surgeon should discuss the surgery with your primary care physician or cardiologist, and you may need to undergo blood testing before your operation. Don't stop taking any medications on your own without consulting your medical doctor or cardiologist.

Inform your eye surgeon if you take or have ever taken an alpha blocker, such as alfuzosin (Uroxatral), doxazosin (Cardura), silodosin (Rapaflo), tamsulosin (Flomax), or terazosin (Hytrin). These drugs are used mainly to treat an enlarged prostate in men, but they may be prescribed for high blood pressure or urinary retention in women. Alpha blockers, along with tolterodine (Detrol) and the herb saw palmetto (both used to treat benign prostate enlargement), can interfere with the medications used to keep your pupils dilated during cataract surgery. By knowing ahead of time that you take one of these drugs, your surgeon can take special steps before or during surgery to avoid complications. Depending on your medical situation, your doctor may prescribe antibiotic eye drops, anti-inflammatory eye drops, or both before the surgery.

During and after surgery

Topical anesthesia (administered directly to the eye in the form of drops, without a needle or injection) or local anesthesia (an injection given by needle around the eye) both prevent pain during surgery. Your surgeon will recommend the type of anesthesia that is best for you. In addition, you will receive light, short-acting sedation through an intravenous line. The entire procedure usually lasts less than half an hour, during which time you may see light, hear noises, and be aware of the surgical team. However, you probably will not see formed images, and you may not be able to tell whether your eye is open or closed.

Afterward, the surgeon may cover the eye with a bandage or shield, which may be removed later that day or the following day. Typically you will be discharged after you rest for a while in the recovery area, but you will need someone to drive you home. Reading and watching television are permitted almost immediately. Although it's a good idea to take it easy, most people can resume normal activities within a few days. Check with your doctor before driving or doing anything strenuous.

Vision usually improves soon after cataract surgery. Some people have excellent vision within hours. Others take several days or even a few weeks to return to normal. This longer interval does not necessarily indicate any complication or failure of the surgery.

During the healing process, you may be surprised at how much brighter colors look. Because the clouded lens (which commonly filters out some colors) has been removed, colors may appear more luminous or seem to have a bluish glow. When you go indoors from bright sunlight, objects may have a reddish afterimage.

Sticky eyelids, itching, sensitivity to light, and mild tearing are perfectly normal after surgery, but severe pain and sudden changes in vision are unusual and warrant an immediate call to your doctor. People who have minor discomfort can take a non-aspirin pain reliever such as acetaminophen (Tylenol) every four to six hours. Any discomfort should subside on its own within a day or two.

Your ophthalmologist will schedule several postoperative visits: the day after surgery, after about a week, and at about a month. It's safest to avoid driving until after your one-day visit, at which time you should ask your doctor about driving. At each visit, the doctor will examine your eye, test your visual acuity, and measure your eye pressure. You probably won't get a new eyeglass prescription until three to six weeks after your surgery.

Self-care

Once at home, you will use antibiotic and cortisone eyedrops, as well as possibly a nonsteroidal anti-inflammatory eye drop, to prevent infection and reduce inflammation. Wash your hands thoroughly before applying the drops, and avoid touching the bottle tip to your eye. Because your eye is more sensitive after surgery, avoid rubbing or touching it. To avoid accidentally rubbing your eye while you sleep, you may need to wear a protective eye shield at night for a few days or weeks.

Your doctor will show you how to clean your eyelids, which may become crusted from discharge. Many people wear medium-density sunglasses when outdoors to screen out glare, even though most implants have ultraviolet blockers (see "Investing in the right sunglasses," page 19).

Make sure you understand all of your doctor's postoperative care instructions. To help ensure a rapid and full recovery, it's important that you follow these instructions carefully. Discuss any questions with your doctor.

Possible complications

More than 98% of people who undergo cataract surgery have improved vision and an uneventful recuperation afterward, assuming they have no other eye disease or serious medical condition. Although cataract surgery is generally very safe, the operation does involve some risk. Fortunately, most complications can be treated with medications, glasses, or a second surgery. The risk of partial or total vision loss is very low. Following are some potential complications of cataract surgery.

Infection of the eye (endophthalmitis). Most ophthalmologists use topical or injected antibiotics before, during, and after surgery to minimize this risk. If you do get an infection (symptoms include red, swollen, painful eyes and vision loss), see your doctor right away.

Swelling and fluid in the center of the retina (cystoid macular edema). Symptoms include blurred or reduced central vision. This can be treated with steroid injections or nonsteroidal anti-inflammatory eyedrops. It's important to take your drops exactly as your doctor prescribed to reduce this risk.

Swelling of the clear covering of the eye (corneal edema). If you have this complication, you'll probably notice blurred vision or haloes around lights. Corneal edema is often temporary, and it can be treated with saline eye drops. If edema doesn't improve and it significantly interferes with your vision

months after surgery (which is unusual), a transplant procedure can be done to replace part or all of your cornea (see "Corneal edema," page 12).

Bleeding in the front or back of the eye (hyphema, vitreous hemorrhage, or suprachoroidal hemorrhage). This is a relatively uncommon complication. Bleeding often clears on its own, but severe bleeding can lead to elevated eye pressure and a loss of vision. Occasionally, a second surgery is needed to clear the bleeding.

Retinal detachment. This rare complication is treated with surgery in the eye doctor's office or hospital operating room (see "Retinal tear or detachment," page 14).

Problems with glare. Glare can be temporary or permanent, but it rarely has serious effects on vision.

Dislocation of the IOL. Shifting of the lens implant is relatively unusual, but it can happen, especially after an eye injury or with certain eye conditions (such as pseudoexfoliation). The dislocation can occur months to years after the procedure. If the dislocation affects your vision, you may need surgery to reposition the lens.

Clouding of the portion of the lens capsule that remains after surgery (posterior capsular opacification, or PCO). This occurs in 30% of patients months to years after their surgery. When PCO affects vision, it can be treated with laser surgery.

Increased pressure in the eye or glaucoma. A rise in pressure is usually temporary. Glaucoma medications can usually control eye pressure (see "Glaucoma," page 29).

Astigmatism. This can be managed with glasses or refractive surgery.

Eye muscle imbalance (strabismus). Problems with the eye muscle can cause cross-eye, the inability of both eyes to focus on the same object at the same time, or double vision. This effect is sometimes temporary. A permanent eye muscle imbalance can be treated with eyeglass modifications (prisms) or, rarely, eye muscle surgery.

Drooping of the upper eyelid (ptosis). If the drooping is severe, it can be treated with lid muscle surgery (see "Ptosis," page 10). ◢

Glaucoma

More than three million Americans have glaucoma, according to the Glaucoma Research Foundation, but about half of them don't know it because typically there are no symptoms in the early stages of the disease. By the year 2030, experts estimate, that number will rise to 4.2 million people.

Glaucoma generally begins by chipping away at peripheral vision and can end by stealing sight entirely. It is a major cause of blindness, accounting for up to 12% of all cases of total vision loss. The problem increases with age. Glaucoma threatens sight in 2% of people over age 40, but up to 10% of those over 80. Early diagnosis and treatment can almost always save vision, which is why regular eye exams are crucial.

What causes glaucoma?

Glaucoma is a group of eye diseases that cause vision loss by damaging the optic nerve. Doctors used to think that high pressure within the eye, called intraocular pressure, was the only cause of this damage. Now they know that other factors besides pressure must be involved, because some susceptible people with normal intraocular pressure also experience vision loss from glaucoma.

Normally, the aqueous humor—the liquid that fills the area just behind the iris—circulates through the pupil into the front compartment of the eye, nourishing the lens and the cells lining the cornea. It then passes through a circular, sieve-like system of tissues called the trabecular meshwork and drains out of the eye through Schlemm's canal. From there, it is absorbed into surrounding blood vessels. The process works continuously. As this clear fluid leaves the eye, fresh aqueous humor is produced to keep a healthy balance of pressure in the eye (see Figure 8, at left).

In glaucoma, this drainage system breaks down, slowing or blocking the outflow of fluid. The fluid backs up in the eye, much like water in a clogged sink, and internal pressure rises. This, in turn, puts stress on the optic nerve. If the pressure continues unabated, nerve fibers that carry optical messages to the brain begin to die off, and vision starts to fade. Obstruction of tiny blood vessels that feed the retina and optic nerve can also lead to vision loss. Nerve fibers on the outer edge of the optic nerve typically die first, affect-

Figure 8: The anatomy of glaucoma

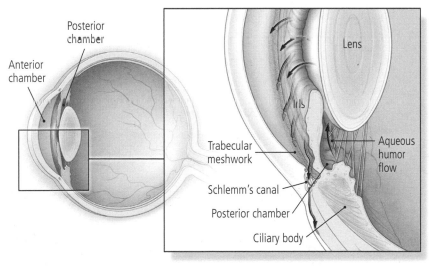

In a healthy eye, the ciliary body continuously produces aqueous humor, a clear liquid that circulates from the posterior chamber into the anterior chamber of the eye and helps maintain its shape and pressure. The fluid (see arrows) bathes and nourishes the tissues at the front of the eye, then drains through the trabecular meshwork into small blood vessels.

If this sieve-like meshwork is blocked, aqueous humor accumulates, and pressure inside the eye increases, causing closed-angle glaucoma. In open-angle glaucoma, the meshwork remains open, but the fluid drains too slowly. In both cases, the excess fluid places undue pressure on the optic nerve in the back of the eye (not shown), and nerve fibers gradually begin to die off, leading to vision loss.

ing peripheral vision (see Figure 9, below right). The damage gradually closes in until the cells supplying central vision are destroyed as well. While optic nerve damage and vision loss from glaucoma are irreversible, there are many effective treatments to prevent both from happening.

While pressure plays an important role in most glaucoma cases, other mechanisms also appear to cause cell death in nerve fibers. Scientists are now investigating ways to prevent this cell death through several different strategies, collectively known as neuroprotection. However, the results of studies on neuroprotective treatments could still be years away.

For now, your best defense against glaucoma is to get screened regularly, starting at age 40 (see "Diagnosing glaucoma," page 32). Start earlier—at age 35—if you have risks like a family history of glaucoma or if you have diabetes. If you catch the disease in its early stages, medications can slow its progress and prevent vision loss.

Another good glaucoma prevention strategy is to exercise for 30 minutes a day, at least five days a week. A study presented at the 2017 American Academy of Ophthalmology annual meeting found that the most physically active participants had a 73% lower risk of developing glaucoma than those who were least active. The faster and more vigorously they exercised, the more their risk dropped.

Types of glaucoma

Although more than two dozen types of glaucoma exist, the following types affect the greatest number of people.

Open-angle glaucoma

This is the most common form of the disease, accounting for more than 90% of all cases. It strikes black and Hispanic people far more frequently than whites, is most prevalent in people over 60, and tends to run in families.

The name comes from the fact that the passage through which fluid drains from the anterior chamber of the eye—located in the angle where the iris meets the cornea—remains open, yet the aqueous humor drains out too slowly, leading to fluid backup and a gradual but persistent elevation in pressure. Consistently uncontrolled high pressure damages the optic nerve and causes vision loss. Because the condition generally has no symptoms in its early stages, regular eye exams are important, especially for anyone at increased risk.

You are at higher risk for open-angle glaucoma if you

- are African American or Hispanic
- are over age 60
- are severely nearsighted or farsighted
- have had an eye injury or eye surgery
- have a family history of the condition
- have thin corneas (see "The importance of corneal thickness," page 31)
- have high intraocular pressure
- use corticosteroid medications.

Several studies also suggest that obstructive sleep apnea—repeated pauses in breathing that occur while you're asleep—can affect blood flow to the optic nerve. Having this condition may increase optic nerve damage in people with all types of glaucoma.

Closed-angle glaucoma

In closed-angle glaucoma, pressure in the eye rises rapidly to as high as 50 to 70 millimeters of mercury

Figure 9: Glaucoma vision

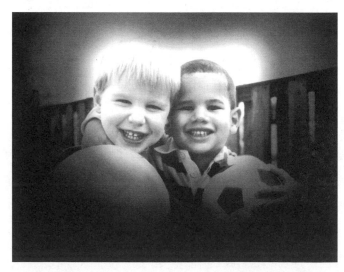

As glaucoma progresses, you may notice that your peripheral vision diminishes.

Photo courtesy of the National Eye Institute.

The importance of corneal thickness

The thickness of your cornea (the clear part of the eye's protective covering) plays a role in the accuracy of your eye pressure reading. The devices that measure pressure rely on flattening the cornea, which is easier to do in people with thinner corneas. Therefore, people with thin corneas (less than 540 micrometers) tend to have artificially low intraocular pressure readings. If your actual pressure is higher than the reading indicates, you might have glaucoma without realizing it. In addition, having a thin cornea is an independent risk factor for glaucoma.

On the flip side, people with thick corneas can have an artificially *high* pressure reading, which could lead to unnecessary treatment.

Fortunately, there is a quick, painless test called pachymetry to measure corneal thickness. This measurement (done routinely with pressure screenings) enables your doctor to obtain a more accurate assessment of your intraocular pressure and develop an appropriate treatment plan.

(mm Hg), versus a normal range of 8 to 21. This occurs when the angle between the iris and cornea narrows and the iris suddenly blocks the trabecular meshwork, preventing fluid from flowing out. When this form of the disorder occurs, the eyeball quickly hardens and the pressure causes pain and blurred vision. Also, people often see halos—colored rings around lights. Closed-angle glaucoma is a medical emergency that must be treated right away to prevent vision loss.

You are at higher risk for closed-angle glaucoma if you

- are Asian
- are farsighted
- are female
- have a shallow anterior chamber or small eye (short axial length).

Low-tension or normal-tension glaucoma

Approximately 30% of people with open-angle glaucoma have eye pressures that fall into the normal range of 8 to 21 mm Hg. Despite the "normal" eye pressure, the optic nerve in these individuals becomes damaged. Symptoms don't usually occur until late in the disease, when blind spots may appear in the peripheral vision. The diagnosis is often made after vision damage has already occurred, but more sensitive diagnostic techniques (optic nerve imaging and visual field testing) are making it possible to detect this disease earlier, before peripheral vision is lost. You can usually stabilize the condition by lowering pressure with medication, surgery, or both.

You are at higher risk for low-tension glaucoma if you have

- abnormal blood flow in the eye
- an autoimmune disease
- low blood pressure
- a disorder that affects blood vessels, such as migraines or Raynaud's phenomenon
- a family history of glaucoma, particularly low-tension glaucoma.

Secondary glaucoma

Secondary glaucoma can develop as a result of some other eye problem—such as chronic inflammation in the eye (uveitis), injury, cataract, diabetes, or a blood vessel blockage in the eye. Rarely, it happens as a complication of cataract surgery. Corticosteroids (oral, inhaled, or topical) can also increase intraocular pressure, especially in people with glaucoma or a family history of glaucoma. People who take these medicines should have their eye doctor carefully monitor their eye pressure.

Symptoms of glaucoma

Open-angle glaucoma is generally a silent disease, with no apparent symptoms in its early stages. Even blind spots or diminishing peripheral vision may not be noticeable until the disease is already advanced. Occasionally, people realize something is awry when they repeatedly need new eyeglass prescriptions or have trouble adjusting to the dark. However, these symptoms generally occur later in the disease. Regular screening is essential, because vision loss is preventable if you discover the condition before the nerve is damaged.

Symptoms of closed-angle glaucoma are much more obvious. Most people experience blurred vision, eye pain, light sensitivity, rainbow halos around lights, headaches, nausea, and vomiting. This serious condition can cause permanent optic nerve damage and even blindness in a matter of hours or days and therefore requires immediate medical attention. If you can't reach your ophthalmologist right away, go to an emergency room.

Diagnosing glaucoma

Regular screening is the best way to prevent glaucoma from stealing your sight (see Table 1, page 17). If you're at risk for glaucoma, get a baseline screening at age 40. After that, get tested once every one to three years. After age 65, increase the frequency to once every six to 12 months. If you have a family history of glaucoma, you should be screened yearly unless you have additional risk factors that mean you should be screened more often. Ask your ophthalmologist for guidance.

During your exam, the ophthalmologist will evaluate your eye pressure using tonometry (see "Measuring eye pressure," page 18). Normal pressure is 8 to 21 mm Hg, but people with eye pressure in this range can still develop the disease (see "Low-tension or normal-tension glaucoma," page 31). Conversely, some people with slightly elevated pressure never develop glaucoma. The amount of stress the optic nerve can withstand differs for each person and each eye. Because eye pressure can vary at different times of day, your doctor may repeat the tonometry test at a different appointment.

The doctor will use both a slit lamp and an oph-

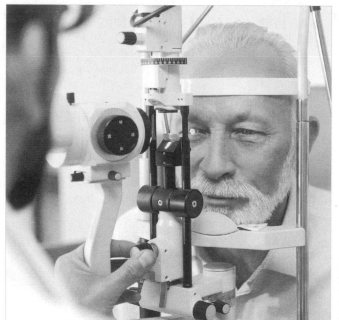

During an eye examination for glaucoma, many types of tests are performed. These tests measure pressure inside the eye, check for problems with the optic nerve, and assess peripheral vision.

thalmoscope to look for any deterioration of your optic nerve. If glaucoma affects the front surface of the nerve (the optic disc), the doctor may see a characteristic called cupping: the disc may appear indented, and its color—normally pinkish yellow—may turn pale and more yellow because the advancing disease has slowed blood flow to the area.

If your eye pressure is not in the normal range or your optic nerve looks unusual, the doctor will perform one or two specialized glaucoma tests:

Visual field test. Also called perimetry, this test requires you to look straight ahead and indicate whether you see tiny specks of light flashing on and off in different locations within your peripheral (side) vision.

Gonioscopy. In this procedure, the doctor places a special contact lens on the surface of your numbed eye. The lens has mirrors and facets that, when studied through the slit lamp, give a detailed view of the corner of your eye and show whether the drainage angle is open, narrowed, or closed.

If you have glaucoma, your ophthalmologist may use a technique called fundus photography to produce three-dimensional pictures of your optic disc. These images will serve as a baseline for later comparisons

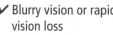

Symptoms of glaucoma

Open-angle glaucoma

✔ Few or no symptoms in early stages

✔ Blind spots and diminishing peripheral vision in later stages

Closed-angle glaucoma
(This is a medical emergency; call your doctor immediately.)

✔ Severe pain

✔ Nausea

✔ Colored halos around lights

✔ Eye redness

✔ Blurry vision or rapid vision loss

of the disc. If the disc changes over time, your pressure hasn't been well controlled and you need more aggressive treatment. Several newer techniques use computer-generated images to analyze the fiber layers of the optic nerve. Over time, these tests can detect the loss of optic nerve fibers, allowing your doctor to track the progression of the disease.

Treating glaucoma

Most types of glaucoma—including open-angle glaucoma, the most common type—can be controlled but not cured. No treatment can restore lost vision, but you can stop the disease from progressing by keeping your pressure under control. Studies have shown that lowering eye pressure prevents optic nerve damage and vision loss in people with all stages of glaucoma—from those who are newly diagnosed to those with advanced disease. Lowering eye pressure can even protect your vision if you don't have glaucoma but your eye pressure is high (ocular hypertension).

For open-angle glaucoma, treatment usually begins with topical medications—eye drops or sometimes ointments—administered one or more times a day (see Table 2, page 34). Depending on the severity of your condition, you might need to use multiple drops or pills. Most ophthalmologists begin with the lowest effective dose to minimize cost and potential side effects.

To apply the drops, tilt your head back while standing and pull your lower lid out to create a small pouch for the medicine. Let the drop fall into the pocket. Gently close your eye to ensure that the medicine spreads over your eye's surface. Try not to blink, squint, or shut your eyes too tightly. These movements could push the drops back out of your eyes.

Although drops can keep your pressure at a safe level, their side effects might prevent you from using them often enough to be effective. Because the drops can enter your bloodstream through your nose and throat, you may have side effects throughout your body (such as a headache or pounding heart)—not just in your eyes. To minimize the amount of medicine that gets into your bloodstream, press your fingertip against the inner corner of your eye for two to three minutes after applying the drops. This compresses the tear duct and prevents the medicine from entering the drainage pathway into your nose.

Follow your doctor's treatment recommendations and take your medications regularly to manage your glaucoma and preserve your vision. If you have questions about your drugs, trouble following your treatment plan, or difficulty using your medicine, ask your doctor for advice.

Regular exams are equally important. Without monitoring, you can't know whether pressure in your eye is in a safe range or if your vision is slowly deteriorating. Each year, people with glaucoma typically

Continued on page 35

Home testing for glaucoma

Regular glaucoma checks from your ophthalmologist are an accurate and effective way to make sure your eye pressure stays under control. But having the ability to test your eye pressure at home could help your doctor better monitor your progress and quickly make adjustments to your medications, if needed.

One home monitoring method that recently gained FDA approval is called iCare Home. In studies, about 75% of people were able to use this device themselves and got results similar to those obtained by ophthalmologists. However, the convenience of home glaucoma monitoring comes at a high cost—over $3,000 to purchase the device—and it isn't currently covered by health insurance. If you want to buy iCare Home, you must do it through your eye doctor, because it isn't sold directly to consumers online or in stores. To learn more about this product, you can download the free iCare Home app to your smartphone.

Researchers at Columbia University are working on a "smart" contact lens, which they say can continuously monitor for changes in eye pressure. The device contains a sensor that detects changes in the curve of the lens that occur with fluctuations in eye pressure. When the device picks up changes, it generates a signal that a wireless device records. When investigators tested the device on 40 patients with open-angle glaucoma, the detection of more signal spikes correlated to faster disease progression.

You can use an online tool to check your peripheral vision. The KeepYourSight Foundation (www.keepyoursight.org) offers a free visual field test called Peristat, which it claims can detect visual field defects to identify glaucoma. Before you use any online test, it's a good idea to check with your ophthalmologist.

Table 2: Glaucoma medications

These drugs are taken topically as eye drops, unless otherwise noted.

GENERIC NAME (BRAND NAME)	DOSES PER DAY	SIDE EFFECTS/COMMENTS
Adrenergics		
dipivefrin* (AKPro, Propine)	2–3	Headache, stinging, redness, burning, temporary blurring of vision. May cause pounding heart and fast heartbeat in some people.
Alpha agonists		
apraclonidine* (Iopidine) brimonidine* (Alphagan)	2–3	Stinging, burning, redness of the eyes, dry mouth, blurred vision, fatigue. Rarely, cardiovascular side effects like a pounding heart.
Beta blockers		
betaxolol* (Betoptic, others) carteolol* (Cartrol, Ocupress) levobetaxolol (Betaxon) levobunolol* (AKBeta, Betagan) metipranolol* (OptiPranolol) timolol maleate* (Betimol, Istalol, Timoptic-XE)	1–2	Stinging, irritation, blurred vision, tearing, allergic reaction. Elderly people are especially prone to side effects. May cause breathing problems in people with asthma. Can slow heart rate in those with heart disease. May cause mental and physical lethargy. Men may experience a decrease in libido.
Carbonic anhydrase inhibitors		
Oral acetazolamide* (Diamox) methazolamide* (Neptazane)	2–3	Dizziness, diarrhea, loss of appetite, metallic taste in the mouth, numbness or tingling in hands and feet, weight loss, fatigue, excessive urination, anemia. Can lead to loss of potassium.
Topical (eye drops) brinzolamide (Azopt) dorzolamide hydrochloride* (Trusopt)	2–3	Burning, stinging, bitter taste in mouth, corneal inflammation, allergic reaction. Dorzolamide is also available in oral form; drops have fewer side effects for most people.
Miotics		
echothiophate (Phospholine Iodide)	3–4	Blurred vision, change in near or distance vision, reduced night vision, headache, eyelid twitching, tearing, sweating, diarrhea.
pilocarpine* (Betoptic Pilo, Isoptic Carpine, Ocusert Pilo, Pilopine HS Gel, others)		Blurred vision, change in near or distance vision, reduced night vision.
Prostaglandins		
bimatoprost* (Lumigan) latanoprost* (Xalatan) tafluprost (Zioptan) travoprost* (Travatan)	1	Burning, stinging, itching, redness, blurred vision. Used only once a day; some people report growth of lashes or change in eye color (the latter resulting from an increase in brown pigment in the iris).
Prostaglandin analog		
latanoprostene bunod (Vyzulta)	1	Redness, irritation, pain, and eyelash growth.
Rho kinase inhibitor		
netarsudil (Rhopressa)	1	Redness, pain, brown or gray deposits in the eye, bleeding, blurry vision, increased tearing, eyelid redness.
Combination medications		
brinzolamide plus brimonidine tartrate (Simbrinza) timolol plus brimonidine (Combigan) timolol plus dorzolamide hydrochloride* (Cosopt)	2	See the individual components, above, to gauge the side effects of these combination products.

Note: Another class of glaucoma medications known as hyperosmotics is used only to control sudden elevations in eye pressure. Hyperosmotics are given orally or by injection; examples include glycerin (Osmoglyn) and isosorbide (Ismotic).

*These medications are available in generic versions.

Continued from page 33

undergo two to four exams to check their visual acuity, optic nerve, and eye pressure. The visual field test and other tests are done at selected intervals to determine whether the disease is stable or if it's worsening—signaling the need for more aggressive treatment.

In some respects, treating glaucoma is like treating heart disease. Managing either condition can require multiple medications. And in both cases, therapy is a lifetime commitment. It's important to stick with your treatment plan even when you don't notice any improvement. Often the benefits are not immediately obvious. Or your medications may need some tweaking. Like blood pressure, intraocular eye pressure varies over the course of the day, so your doctor may tailor your medication schedule to address daily eye pressure fluctuations.

Overcoming obstacles to using your drops

Glaucoma eye drops are very effective, but they won't protect your sight if you don't use them. Studies show that more than half of people with this disease don't stick to their treatment regimen, often because they have difficulty applying their eye drops. If you're struggling to get the drops into your eyes, ask your ophthalmologist to talk you through the process. Or, use one of several assistive devices. For example, an eye drop guide attaches to the medicine bottle. It holds your eye open and focuses the drop straight into your eye. If you have arthritis or other mobility issues, you can buy an automated bottle squeezer to make it easier to squeeze out the drops.

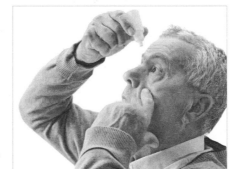

If the high cost of your prescriptions is standing in the way of treatment, a number of patient assistance programs are available to help you pay for your medications. These include

- GoodRx (www.goodrx.com)
- The Medicine Program (www.themedicineprogram.com)
- NeedyMeds (www.needymeds.org)
- Partnership for Prescription Assistance (www.pparx.org)
- RetailMeNot RxSaver (www.lowestmed.com)
- Rx Assist (www.rxassist.org).

It is also important to talk to your ophthalmologist about the high cost of your medications, as there may be alternatives.

Glaucoma medications

Glaucoma drug development has been ongoing since the 1990s, but only recently have any new drugs been introduced. In 2017, the FDA approved two glaucoma drugs—the first truly novel glaucoma medications in 20 years.

One is latanoprostene bunod (Vyzulta), which, like the prostaglandins, lowers eye pressure by increasing the flow of fluid out of the eye through nearby tissues, in addition to the conventional route of the angle and the trabecular meshwork. *Unlike* the prostaglandins, Vyzulta has a second mechanism of action. It lowers eye pressure by releasing nitric oxide, which relaxes the trabecular meshwork and makes it work more efficiently.

The other new glaucoma drug, netarsudil (Rhopressa), works in an entirely novel way through so-called rho-associated protein kinase inhibitors, or ROCK inhibitors, which block enzymes that control cellular structures involved in cell shape and movements. ROCK inhibitors are thought to lower eye pressure by relaxing the trabecular meshwork and Schlemm's canal. This decreases the resistance to drainage through the conventional outflow pathway, thus lowering eye pressure.

Following is a list of both the older and newer medications, presented in the order in which an ophthalmologist is most likely to prescribe them. However, the doctor will adjust treatment to your individual needs. Depending on the severity of your glaucoma and your medical history, your doctor may prescribe these drugs in a different order or use two or more drugs in combination. The more commonly used medications tend to have fewer and less severe side effects than those that are prescribed less often (see Table 2, page 34). Remember that drugs are only helpful if you use them (see "Overcoming obstacles to using your drops," at left).

Prostaglandins. Many people use prostaglandin eye drops because these drugs require only one application per day. Prostaglandins lower eye pressure by increasing the flow of aqueous humor through the uveal and scleral tissues rather than through the trabecular meshwork.

Beta blockers. These eye drops contain medication similar to the beta blockers used to treat some types of heart disease. Beta blockers lower pressure in the eye by reducing the amount of aqueous humor produced by the ciliary body. This class of medication is usually well tolerated, but side effects may occur. You can use beta blocker eye drops even if you are also taking beta blockers in pill form for heart disease, but you should notify both your ophthalmologist and cardiologist or primary care doctor that you are doing so.

Carbonic anhydrase inhibitors. Medications in this class, also known as CAIs, can be used either orally or topically to decrease eye pressure. They work by reducing the amount of aqueous humor produced in the eye.

Alpha agonists. These eye drops lower pressure in the eye by both decreasing production of aqueous humor and increasing fluid outflow.

Adrenergics. These eye drops reduce the amount of aqueous humor and increase its outflow through the trabecular meshwork.

Miotics. These are the oldest of the current glaucoma medications. Applied as eye drops, they improve drainage of fluid through the trabecular meshwork. Miotics are not used as often as they once were because they have more side effects than newer drugs—including dim vision at night or in darkened rooms.

Rho kinase inhibitor. The first eyedrop for glaucoma in this class is netarsudil (Rhopressa). When taken once a day, it works by increasing the flow of aqueous humor out of the trabecular meshwork.

Dual-mechanism prostaglandin analog and nitric oxide stimulator. The first eyedrop for glaucoma in this class is latanoprostene bunod (Vyzulta). When taken once a day, this medication enhances fluid outflow through both the trabecular meshwork and other tissues in order to lower intraocular pressure.

Hyperosmotics. Hyperosmotic medications are used in oral or intravenous form for severely elevated eye pressure in glaucoma. They quickly reduce pressure in the eye by pulling fluid from the eyeball into the blood vessels inside the eye. The fluid then leaves the eye with the normal blood flow.

Potential new drugs. Researchers are currently investigating new treatments (both eyedrops and oral medication) to lower eye pressure. Some therapies under development improve the function of retinal ganglion cells—the nerve cells that transmit visual information from the eye to the brain. Other potential new therapies protect the optic nerve through various mechanisms.

Figure 10: Laser trabeculoplasty for glaucoma

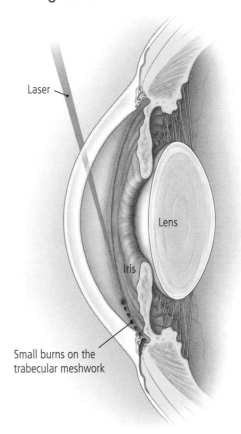

In this procedure, the surgeon uses a laser to produce small burns on the trabecular meshwork. The light energy tightens the beams of the trabecular meshwork, creating more space between them and thereby increasing the flow of aqueous humor out of the eye. It also causes metabolic changes in the drainage system by recruiting macrophages (a type of white blood cell) and other cells that enhance the activity of the drain. The results begin to wane within several years, at which time the procedure might need to be repeated or medications adjusted or added.

Glaucoma surgery

If medication fails to control your eye pressure, your ophthalmologist may recommend either laser or incisional glaucoma surgery.

Laser trabeculoplasty. This procedure uses highly focused light energy from lasers to treat open-angle glaucoma (see Figure 10, page 36). There are two versions: argon laser trabeculoplasty and selective laser trabeculoplasty. Both treatments lower eye pressure more than 75% of the time.

Laser trabeculoplasty is done in an ophthalmologist's office, and it usually takes less than 10 minutes. After you receive anesthetic drops to numb your eye, the doctor puts a temporary contact lens on your eye, then focuses and applies the laser. You may see flashes of green or red light during the procedure, but you won't feel any pain. The doctor then checks your eye pressure and prescribes anti-inflammatory eye drops for you to use at home. You may experience blurred vision and sensitivity to light for a day or two after the operation, but real discomfort is rare. You'll probably still need to keep taking your regular glaucoma medicines after the procedure.

Laser trabeculoplasty is often helpful, but the benefits may not be permanent. As the treatment effect wanes (usually within two to three years), you may need additional medicines or more surgery.

Laser iridotomy. Doctors use this procedure to treat people who have closed-angle glaucoma or are at risk for it. Like trabeculoplasty, this procedure is done in an ophthalmologist's office. After numbing your eye and applying a temporary contact lens to guide the laser, the doctor creates a tiny hole—no bigger than the head of a pin—in your iris. The new hole prevents blockage of fluid behind the iris and allows fluid to drain internally through the trabecular meshwork of the eye. This restores the balance between fluid entering and leaving your eye and stabilizes eye pressure. The procedure takes only a few minutes. Laser iridotomy often cures closed-angle glaucoma. Occasionally, people who have this procedure need additional treatment with medications or incisional surgery.

Incisional glaucoma surgery. If medications or laser treatment don't lower your eye pressure enough, of if you are not a candidate for laser surgery, you may need incisional surgery. Following are the options.

- **Glaucoma filtration surgery (trabeculectomy)** is the most common type of incisional surgery. This delicate microsurgical procedure is done in an operating room under local anesthesia. The eye surgeon makes a small flap in the sclera (the white of the eye) where it meets the cornea (the clear covering over the lens and iris). A window opening is then created under the flap to remove a portion of the sclera, Schlemm's canal, and the trabecular meshwork. A small hole cut in the iris (iridectomy) will prevent future blockage. The doctor closes the flap with several tiny stitches. Next, the membrane covering the sclera (the conjunctiva) is closed in a watertight manner to form a reservoir (filtration bleb). The aqueous humor inside the eye can then drain through the flap to collect in the reservoir, where it is absorbed by blood vessels and other nearby tissues. Some of the stitches may be removed after surgery to increase fluid drainage and lower the pressure inside your eye. You will likely receive medications to help reduce scarring in your eye both during and after surgery.

- **Shunts.** If your doctor is concerned that a trabeculectomy will not be successful, he or she may recommend an aqueous shunt. This is a small plate with a tube. The doctor places the plate under the conjunctiva and sews it to the sclera, then inserts the tube into the anterior chamber. The shunt drains excess fluid into a reservoir around the plate.

- **Stents.** Another option is to implant a stent—a small titanium tube—in the meshwork between the iris and cornea to improve fluid drainage and decrease eye pressure.

Incisional surgery helps to lower eye pressure in many people, allowing them to reduce or even stop taking their glaucoma medications. However, up to 20% of people need a second surgery. The reservoirs created by this surgery may leak, become infected, or fail to form. Incisional surgery may also lead to blurred or reduced vision or the development of a cataract.

Laser cyclophotocoagulation. This outpatient procedure treats several types of glaucoma, including open- and closed-angle glaucoma. Your doctor might recommend laser cyclophotocoagulation if a previous surgical procedure didn't control your pressure. A laser is aimed at the ciliary body, the structure behind the iris that produces aqueous humor, to help reduce the amount of fluid entering the eye. This, in turn, lowers eye pressure. The procedure is often performed at the same time as cataract surgery. It can also be done endoscopically, using a miniature camera to view the treatment area. This allows for much more precise direction of the laser beam and leads to fewer complications. Although serious complications are rare, this surgery can cause inflammation, and it may increase the risk of a cataract.

Newer surgical options. A number of new, minimally invasive surgical procedures lower intraocular pressure in a variety of ways. While these procedures are typically done in combination with cataract surgery, some of them can be done as stand-alone glaucoma surgery. These procedures are often referred to by the names of the devices that are used to perform them.

- **Canaloplasty** uses a small incision to widen the eye's drainage canal, allowing more aqueous fluid to drain out.
- **Deep sclerotomy** involves making a tiny incision into the sclera to provide a new drainage route.
- **Ex-Press mini shunt** is a small steel device used during the trabeculectomy procedure to reduce the risk of excessively low eye pressure—a possible complication of glaucoma surgery.
- **iStent,** a tiny titanium device implanted during cataract surgery, creates a permanent opening in the trabecular meshwork to improve the flow of fluid from your eyes and control eye pressure. Because it doesn't lower eye pressure as much as procedures like trabeculectomy, iStent is recommended for people who are in the early to moderate stages of glaucoma.
- **Microtrabeculectomy** is an updated version of trabeculectomy surgery that places tiny tubes into the eye to drain fluid. Devices like the Xen Gel Stent and InnFocus Microshunt have been shown in studies to lower pressure effectively, with fewer complications than traditional trabeculectomy. The Xen Gel Stent received FDA approval in 2016. The InnFocus Microshunt is awaiting approval.
- **Trabectome** is a device that uses an electric current to remove tissue from the trabecular meshwork and open up the drainage system. During cataract surgery, the surgeon inserts the device into the eye through the same small corneal incision used to remove the cataract. The tip of this device contains electrodes that burn off sections of tissue in the trabecular meshwork. Studies show the procedure reduces eye pressure by about 30% and reduces the number of eye drops needed. Side effects are minimal. They include blood in the eye after the procedure, which should clear up quickly.
- **Viscocanalostomy** involves inserting a gel-like material called viscoelastic into Schlemm's canal. This improves drainage and lowers eye pressure.

Many of these procedures are still being studied to confirm their effectiveness and safety over time. ◆

Age-related macular degeneration

Unlike glaucoma, which first affects peripheral vision, age-related macular degeneration (AMD) affects central vision. It strikes at the macula—the small central part of the retina that is responsible for sharp images at the center of your visual field. People with AMD often develop blurred or distorted vision and cannot clearly see objects directly in front of them. Eventually they may develop a blind spot in the middle of their field of vision that increases in size as the disease progresses (see Figure 11, below right).

Up to 11 million Americans have AMD, and by the year 2050 that number is expected to double to nearly 22 million. AMD is the leading cause of vision loss in adults ages 60 and older.

Types of AMD

The disease occurs in two main forms: dry and wet. While this report focuses on these two age-related forms, younger people can develop other kinds of macular degeneration, some inherited and some acquired, which may have similarities to age-related macular degeneration.

Dry AMD

The vast majority (90%) of people with AMD have the dry or atrophic type. This form of the disease is caused by a breakdown or thinning of retinal tissue and, in its advanced stages, by the loss of photoreceptor (light-sensitive) cells in the macular area of the retina. The symptoms of dry AMD become more pronounced as the condition progresses. Although some people have no symptoms and are completely unaware that they have the disease, others completely lose their central vision.

Dry AMD has three stages—early, intermediate, and advanced. In the early stage, central vision is usually not affected, though there may be some small abnormalities. In the intermediate phase, a blind spot and blurring may appear. After five years of living with intermediate dry AMD, you are more likely to develop advanced dry AMD, in which the blurring becomes more pronounced, making it hard to read or even recognize people. Dry AMD may affect only one eye at first. It is likely that the second eye is also affected without showing symptoms. The disease may continue to develop in the second eye, and symptoms can appear over time.

Wet AMD

Wet AMD is the advanced, quickly progressive form of the disease that is most likely to cause severe vision loss. Everyone with wet AMD starts out with the dry form. However, only a small percentage of those with dry AMD will go on to develop the wet form. Wet AMD develops when abnormal blood vessels form in the layer of cells beneath the retina (the choroid layer) and extend like tentacles under and into the retina, often toward the macula. These new vessels are prone

Figure 11: Age-related macular degeneration vision

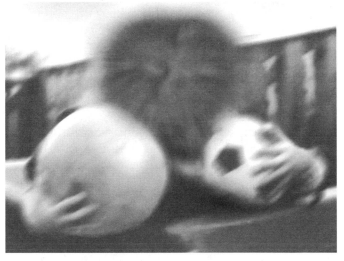

As age-related macular degeneration progresses, you may notice a blind spot develop in your central vision.

Photo courtesy of the National Eye Institute.

to leaking fluid and blood, which damage tissue and photoreceptor cells. The result is scarring and significant vision loss, usually in the center of the macula.

Causes and risk factors

The causes of AMD are not well understood. Scientists don't know exactly why the macula deteriorates. They do know that certain factors can increase your risk of developing AMD.

Aging. People in their 50s have only a 2% chance of developing any form of AMD. That risk jumps to 30% after age 75.

Gender. Women get the disorder more often than men, possibly because they live longer.

Race. White people are more likely to get AMD, and to lose their vision from it, than people of other races.

Smoking. Smokers are up to four times more likely to develop the later stages of macular degeneration. Quitting lowers your risk, with benefits becoming evident after a year of being smoke-free.

Other factors that may increase your risk include

- coronary artery disease
- unprotected exposure to bright sunlight and ultraviolet radiation
- family history of AMD
- farsightedness
- high blood pressure
- high cholesterol
- light-colored eyes
- nighttime drop in blood pressure
- obesity
- sleep apnea.

There has been some question as to whether cataract surgery may play a role in the development of AMD, particularly because many older adults have both conditions. However, research hasn't supported this idea.

The link between diet and AMD has more evidence behind it. Studies have found that AMD is more common in people whose diets are deficient in nutrients such as vitamins C and E, the mineral zinc, and lutein and zeaxanthin (substances known as carotenoids that are found in green leafy vegetables and fruits, and which are the dominant pigments in the macula). A diet high in refined carbohydrates, saturated fat, and sugary foods such as cakes, cookies, and white bread may also raise the risk of AMD.

Ongoing research continues to focus on causes—such as genes, diet, and environmental conditions—with the hope of ultimately preventing AMD. Researchers have identified several gene variants that are linked to a higher risk for AMD, including the complement factor H gene. A few genetic tests for AMD are commercially available. However, the American Academy of Ophthalmology doesn't currently recommend gene testing for AMD. With no real preventive therapies currently available, testing can't do much, if anything, to change the disease course. Genetic information may be more valuable in the future, as newer and more personalized treatment options emerge.

Diagnosing AMD

Often there are no symptoms in the early stages of the disease. As AMD progresses, people with the dry form will have blurred vision and difficulty reading

What is a macular hole?

A macular hole is different from and less common than macular degeneration. It occurs when the vitreous humor, the gel-like substance that fills the back of the eye, pulls away from the surface of the retina, creating traction that may cause a hole to develop in the macula. A person with the severe form of this condition will lose much of his or her central vision.

Ophthalmologists use a procedure called vitrectomy and membrane stripping with gas injection to close the hole and help restore vision. The doctor removes the vitreous humor to prevent it from pulling on the retina, along with any visible scar tissue, and fills the space left behind with a gas bubble. If you have this procedure, you must spend a few days to a week in a face-down position, to allow the gas bubble to push against and gradually seal the hole at the back of the eye. This procedure is more than 90% effective in closing the hole, but the degree of vision improvement varies widely from person to person. Outcomes are best when the surgery is performed early in the course of the disease (typically within the first few months), although vision can improve when it's done anytime within one year.

or distinguishing faces. These can also be symptoms of early-stage wet AMD. Wet AMD typically progresses swiftly if left untreated, causing a blind spot at the center of vision. Over time, this area may enlarge and hinder sight. However, some people who have AMD in only one eye often do not realize they have any vision loss because their healthy eye compensates so well.

Distorted vision is another early sign of wet AMD. Leaking blood vessels raise the position of the macula and cause straight lines to suddenly appear wavy and shapes to look deformed. Colors may seem faded. While AMD can severely damage central vision, it does not affect peripheral vision, and people do not go totally blind from even the most severe forms of the disease.

A routine dilated eye examination can often detect signs of AMD before sight is affected and permanent visual loss occurs. The eye exam includes an acuity test to measure how well you see at different distances (with glasses, if needed). A complete eye exam will rule out or identify coexisting eye diseases, such as cataract or glaucoma.

A doctor may suspect dry AMD if the view through an ophthalmoscope reveals clumps of pigment or clusters of drusen (small yellow deposits that build up under the macula). Although these lesions can indicate early or intermediate stages of dry AMD, drusen alone are not conclusive evidence that you have the disease. If your doctor suspects you have wet AMD, you may undergo additional tests to confirm the diagnosis and help determine the best course of treatment.

Fluorescein angiography. A special dye is injected into your arm. As the dye travels through the blood vessels in the retina, your doctor uses a special camera to take pictures. These images reveal whether the blood vessels in your eyes are leaking, and where any abnormalities are located.

Indocyanine green (ICG). This test uses another injected dye to view the blood circulation in your retina and look for signs of retinal disease.

Optical coherence tomography (OCT). This test uses an ultrasound to take pictures of your retina. It can show fluid in the retina—a sign of wet AMD.

▶ Symptoms of AMD

- ✔ Blurred vision
- ✔ Distorted vision
- ✔ Faded colors
- ✔ Difficulty reading
- ✔ Difficulty distinguishing faces
- ✔ Blind spot in the center of your visual field

Monitoring AMD

The earlier you catch the progression to wet AMD, the greater the likelihood of successful treatment. That's why it's important for everyone with dry AMD to get in the habit of checking their central vision at home at least once a week.

A good way to do this is with the Amsler grid test (see Figure 12, page 42). You focus your eyes on a central dot on a grid that resembles graph paper. If the lines near the dot appear wavy or are missing, you may have AMD. (You can simulate this test by looking at windowpanes, floor tiles, or ceiling tiles to see if the straight edges look wavy.) If you already have dry AMD, it's a good idea to perform this test regularly to check for signs of progression to the wet form of the disease. Distortion on the grid may be a sign of wet AMD and should be evaluated, especially if this distortion is new for you. You can find the Amsler grid and instructions for using it online (www.preventblindness.org/amsler-grid-instructions), or download an app on your smartphone.

A relatively new system called ForeseeHome allows you to monitor changes in AMD at home. Looking into a mounted device with an eyepiece, you will see a succession of straight, dotted lines. When you notice a wave or bump in a line, you click on it using a mouse. It is recommended that you do this at least three to four times per week; it takes about three minutes per eye. A monitoring center assesses the results, and if it detects any changes in your vision, it alerts your doctor so that you can schedule an appointment. Medicare and many private insurance companies cover the cost. Otherwise, you must pay a one-time activation fee and a monthly monitoring fee. In a large, government-sponsored study, people who used ForeseeHome were more likely to detect conversion to wet AMD earlier, resulting in better vision and fewer symptoms, compared with those who relied on conventional monitoring. Research shows that in general, the better your vision is when you start treatment, the better your outcome.

Treating dry AMD

Currently, the only treatment for dry AMD is a well-balanced diet that includes leafy green vegetables—combined with supplements of vitamins studied in the Age-Related Eye Disease Study (AREDS). This study found that daily high doses of vitamins C and E, beta carotene, and the minerals zinc and copper can slow (and sometimes even prevent) progression from intermediate to advanced AMD, thereby preserving vision in many people (see "Vitamins for AMD," page 43).

A follow-up study, AREDS2, sought to determine whether the formulation might be improved by adding omega-3 fatty acids, lutein, and zeaxanthin; removing beta carotene; or reducing zinc. In this subsequent study, adding lutein and zeaxanthin didn't affect the further development (progression) of AMD, but these antioxidants were safer than beta carotene for smokers and people who recently stopped smoking, and

they were particularly helpful for people who were deficient in these carotenoids. For nonsmokers, these supplements may have a modest benefit in reducing progression to advanced AMD.

Although several treatments are available for wet AMD, the dry form of the disease has been harder to conquer. In particular, researchers have focused on slowing what's known as geographic atrophy, the most advanced stage of dry AMD, in which sections of retinal cells die and waste away. Several once-promising drugs have failed to slow the progression of this disease, and have since been shelved, but a few others are still in development. One such drug, APL-2, is in late-stage trials. It's a complement C3 inhibitor, which targets the so-called complement cascade—a series of processes through which the immune system attacks the retina in AMD. In studies conducted so far, the drug slowed the rate of geographic atrophy by nearly 30% compared with a placebo (dummy pill).

Researchers are also investigating whether stem cell therapy can prevent damage to retinal cells in dry AMD. Teams at several research institutes are studying the use of stem cells to regenerate a damaged layer of cells in the back of the eye called the retinal

Figure 12: When central vision is damaged

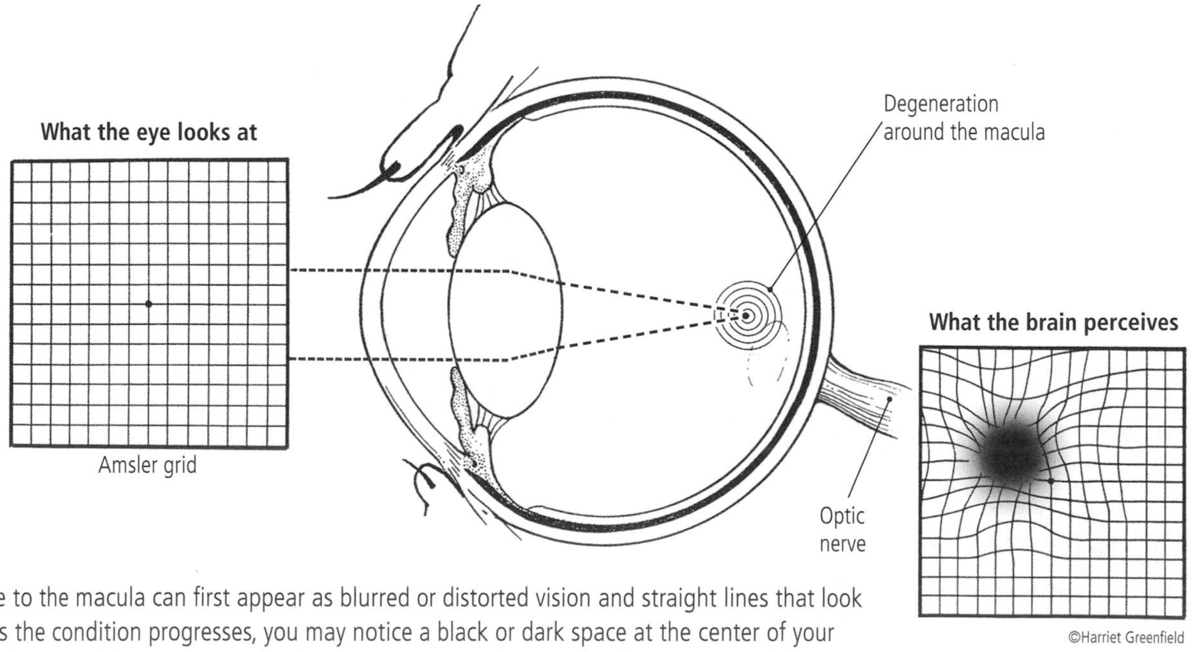

What the eye looks at

Amsler grid

Degeneration around the macula

Optic nerve

What the brain perceives

©Harriet Greenfield

Damage to the macula can first appear as blurred or distorted vision and straight lines that look wavy. As the condition progresses, you may notice a black or dark space at the center of your visual field. An ophthalmologist will ask you to focus on a dot on a grid (called an Amsler grid). If the lines near the dot appear wavy, you could have macular degeneration.

pigment epithelium (see "On the horizon," page 45). The destruction of these cells in AMD contributes to vision loss from the disease.

Because dry AMD progresses very slowly, people are usually able to manage well in their daily routines, even with some central vision loss. If the condition worsens, special low-vision aids—such as magnifying lenses or devices that "read" regular print and then enlarge it on a monitor—can help maintain quality of life (see "Living with low vision," page 50).

Treating wet AMD

Treatment for wet AMD centers on a class of medications known as anti-VEGF drugs. Laser treatment was occasionally used before anti-VEGF therapy, but it is very rarely used today.

Anti-VEGF drugs

Vascular endothelial growth factor (VEGF) is a substance that stimulates the growth of new blood vessels. VEGF has been linked to abnormal blood vessel growth and leakage in AMD and other common retinal diseases, such as diabetic retinopathy and retinal venous occlusive disease. Anti-VEGF drugs block the effects of VEGF (see Figure 13, page 44), inhibiting the growth of abnormal new blood vessels.

To administer anti-VEGF treatment, the doctor first numbs your eye and then injects the drug into your eyeball with a very fine needle. Most people who receive the injection say either it doesn't hurt or it causes mild to moderate discomfort that feels a bit like touching their eye in search of a lost contact lens. You will need injections at regular intervals for several months to several years. Possible side effects include short-term eye pain, irritation, discharge, and seeing spots or floaters, but these are often mild. More serious side effects, including infections that can lead to vision loss, occur in less than one in 2,000 to 3,000 injections.

Three anti-VEGF drugs are FDA-approved for treating wet AMD. Doctors rarely prescribe the oldest one, pegaptanib (Macugen) because the newer drugs—ranibizumab (Lucentis) and aflibercept (Eylea)—are far more effective. A fourth drug, bev-acizumab (Avastin), is FDA-approved for treating several types of cancer, but it has long been used off-label to treat AMD.

Research suggests that Lucentis, Eylea, and Avastin are all highly effective for AMD. Avastin and Lucentis have gone head-to-head in a number of studies, and the two drugs appear to work equally well at stabilizing or improving visual acuity. For some people, one drug might work better than another.

The main difference between these drugs is the cost, which runs about $60 to $70 per dose for Avastin versus up to $2,000 per dose for Lucentis and Eylea. Check your insurance plan or Medicare coverage to see how much of the cost you will need to shoulder (if any) if you choose this therapy.

Because anti-VEGF medications act on blood vessels, some doctors have voiced concerns that these drugs might increase the risk for strokes and other vascular events. Although the long-term safety of anti-VEGF drugs hasn't yet been fully established, so far studies haven't found a marked increase in adverse cardiovascular events.

People with AMD may soon have another treatment option, as a new anti-VEGF therapy is in the drug pipeline. Brolucizumab is currently in phase 3 trials—the last stage of the drug testing process. One advantage it could have over other drugs in this class is its dosing schedule. Eylea and Lucentis are given monthly in the beginning (during the "loading

▶ **Vitamins for AMD**

The clinical trial known as AREDS2 found that a specific combination of antioxidants, zinc, and other nutrients may help protect against advanced age-related macular degeneration:

- vitamin C: 500 milligrams (mg)
- vitamin E: 400 international units (IU)
- zinc: 25 mg
- copper (cupric oxide): 2 mg
- lutein: 10 mg
- zeaxanthin: 2 mg
- omega-3 fatty acids (DHA and EPA): 1,000 mg.

Ask your doctor or pharmacist about the different AREDS study formulations and which one might be right for you.

phase"), after which Lucentis is given once a month, and Eylea, every other month (if used according to the label). By contrast, brolucizumab may be given at three-month intervals after the loading phase in as many as half of patients.

Despite the progress made with anti-VEGF therapies, researchers still haven't been able to overcome one major hurdle in AMD treatment—the need for injections into the eye. A few research teams are investigating more patient-friendly drug delivery methods.

One of the simplest ways to administer these drugs would be with eye drops. Yet topical drops tested so far haven't had much success, largely because of the difficulty in penetrating to the back of the eye. Despite the results to date, topical AMD drugs remain under investigation.

Also being studied is a sustained delivery system for Lucentis. The port delivery system (PDS) is a device pre-filled with the drug that the doctor inserts through the patient's sclera into the vitreous cavity. The device slowly releases Lucentis into the eye over a period of several months or longer. If the PDS receives FDA approval, patients would return periodically to their doctor for a refill, but they could avoid the repeat injections currently required to treat wet AMD.

Gene therapies are also under investigation. For example, researchers are investigating whether a genetic product injected into the eye can induce a patient's cells to produce a substance similar to anti-VEGF drugs that prevents vital cells from becoming damaged (see "On the horizon," page 45).

Laser treatments

Laser surgery is another possible—though uncommon—treatment option for wet AMD. It has lost ground to anti-VEGF drugs because it has two big drawbacks: it often fails to prevent the growth of new blood vessels, and it can destroy both diseased sections of the retina and adjacent healthy ones. Moreover, laser surgery does nothing to correct or slow the underlying disease process in wet AMD.

In general, lasers are used only in situations where the leaking blood vessels are relatively small and located far from the central portion of the macula, or when someone cannot have intraocular injections because of an eye infection or advanced glaucoma. Few people fall into these categories.

When laser surgery is performed, the following treatments can be used.

Laser photocoagulation. In this procedure, the doctor aims a laser at leaky blood vessels to seal them and prevent further seepage. People reap the most benefits when the procedure is done on newly formed vessels that haven't yet encroached on the fovea (the central part of the macula, which provides the clearest vision). Such cases are rare, however, as most people with wet AMD already have blood ves-

Figure 13: Targets for anti-VEGF therapy

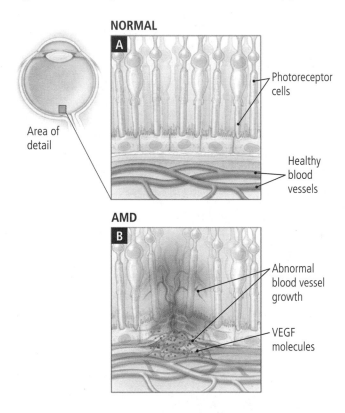

NORMAL
A
Photoreceptor cells
Area of detail
Healthy blood vessels

AMD
B
Abnormal blood vessel growth
VEGF molecules

The wet form of age-related macular degeneration injures healthy tissue in the retina. The top illustration (**A**) shows the blood vessels and photoreceptor cells of a healthy eye. When VEGF molecules stimulate abnormal blood vessel development, blood vessels sprout tentacles that extend under and into the retina, often involving the macula (**B**).

These new vessels are fragile, often leaking blood and other fluids that injure nearby tissues and photoreceptor cells. Anti-VEGF drugs counteract the action of VEGF molecules by inhibiting blood vessel proliferation. These drugs also decrease the amount of leakage from abnormal blood vessels.

sels adjacent to or under the fovea. In people who qualify for the procedure, sealing off the leaking blood vessels may restore vision. Laser photocoagulation can be done in a doctor's office and takes only a few minutes, although sometimes multiple treatments are necessary. You may experience some mild discomfort and sensitivity to light afterward. The surgery is often helpful, but about half of people who have it see a return of symptoms and may need more laser treatments.

Photodynamic therapy. This treatment uses a laser in combination with the light-activated drug verteporfin (Visudyne). The two-step, 15-minute procedure can be done in a doctor's office. First, the drug is injected into a vein in the arm through an intravenous line over a 10-minute period. During the next five minutes, the drug travels through the body and accumulates in the abnormal blood vessels in the eye. The doctor then activates the drug by shining a low-intensity laser into the eye for about 90 seconds. This produces a highly energized form of oxygen that kills abnormally growing cells, closing off the abnormal blood vessels without damaging surrounding healthy eye tissue. For two to five days after Visudyne therapy, your eyes may be especially sensitive to light. You'll also need to avoid exposing your skin or eyes to direct sunlight or bright light. Visudyne therapy alone rarely restores vision; more often, it simply slows retinal damage and vision loss. To preserve vision, people usually need more than one Visudyne treatment per year.

For people who don't get good results from anti-VEGF drugs, doctors sometimes add photodynamic therapy and steroid injections. However, studies have not found that this combination treatment is any more effective than anti-VEGF drugs alone.

On the horizon

At the forefront of AMD research are two breakthrough technologies: gene therapy and stem cell therapy. Although both are still highly preliminary, they could one day provide important new approaches to treatment.

Gene therapy for AMD involves introducing a new gene into the body to control blood vessel growth and improve vision. The doctor uses a virus—similar to the one that causes colds, but modified so that it does not cause disease—to carry a new gene into the eye. The gene codes for a protein that turns cells of the retina into tiny drug-manufacturing plants, producing therapeutic proteins that stop the growth of abnormal blood vessels in much the same way the anti-VEGF drugs ranibizumab (Lucentis) and aflibercept (Eylea) do. A small study published in *The Lancet* showed such an approach was safe, and it decreased the need for injections in at least some of the participants.

Another avenue of research aims to replace damaged retinal cells using stem cells—fledgling cells that can develop into many different kinds of cells in the body. Researchers are examining the potential of embryonic stem cells to replace damaged retinal pigment epithelial cells, which are essential for a healthy retina. Once implanted, stem cells can also release substances called trophic factors, which help the damaged tissue heal and restore itself. In separate trials presented at the 2017 American Academy of Ophthalmology meeting, researchers from Israel and Florida were successfully able to replace AMD-damaged cells with

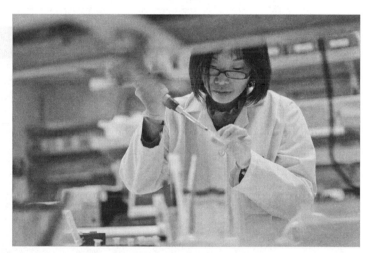

Gene therapy could one day help people with AMD. New genes introduced into the eye can cause the retina to start manufacturing proteins resembling anti-VEGF drugs.

stem cells. The treatment appeared to be safe, and patients' vision remained stable or even improved.

Stem cell therapy is considered controversial, however, because embryonic stem cells are taken from unimplanted human embryos. Also, there is concern that the stem cells might replicate uncontrollably, potentially leading to the development of cancer. So far, research has not shown evidence of this risk.

A great deal of research will be required before such therapies can be proven safe and effective enough to be approved for use in patients outside of clinical trials.

Self-care

Although AMD is not curable, early detection and treatment can prevent damage to the retina. For this reason, it's crucial to have regular eye exams. Because all the available treatments for wet AMD work best in the disease's early stages, consult an ophthalmologist immediately if you notice any vision changes.

People who are already diagnosed with AMD can monitor their condition by testing themselves at home with an Amsler grid (see Figure 12, page 42) or the ForeseeHome monitor (see "Monitoring AMD," page 41). Keep the Amsler grid on the refrigerator door or in another convenient spot. Routine testing can warn someone with dry AMD that wet AMD is beginning, or alert people who already had laser surgery for AMD that blood vessels in the eye are leaking or bleeding.

If you have already lost some of your vision to AMD, low-vision aids can help maximize the sight you have left (see "Living with low vision," page 50). Specialists in low vision can prescribe appropriate aids and refer you to agencies that offer support and assistance to the visually impaired.

Preventing and slowing AMD

While there is no surefire way to prevent AMD, you can take steps to delay the disease or reduce its severity. Because smoking can accelerate AMD damage, quitting smoking is an important preventive step. Wearing a hat and sunglasses that block the sun's blue wavelengths may also provide protection, since blue wavelengths may contribute to the development of AMD.

Evidence also suggests that certain nutrients help prevent macular degeneration. Middle-aged and older people may benefit from diets high in fresh fruits and dark-green leafy vegetables—such as spinach, collard greens, and kale—that are rich in lutein and zeaxanthin.

As for supplements, people at high risk of developing the advanced stages of wet AMD may lower their risk about 25% by taking high-dose combinations of antioxidant vitamins and minerals (see "Vitamins for AMD," page 43). However, supplements don't seem to benefit people who either do not have AMD or who have early AMD. Ask your doctor about taking antioxidant-zinc supplements if you have intermediate or advanced dry AMD or wet AMD.

The omega-3s tested in the AREDS2 formula didn't seem to slow AMD progression, but eating fish and other foods high in these nutrients may still be worthwhile for preserving optimal vision and overall good health. ◆

Diabetic retinopathy

With diabetes turning into a nationwide epidemic, the related eye problem known as diabetic retinopathy has become a serious public health issue. In fact, it's the leading cause of new blindness cases in adults. Nearly eight million Americans live with diabetic retinopathy, and their vision is at risk.

Diabetes comes in two main forms: type 1 and type 2. Type 1 diabetes is an autoimmune disease. The body's own immune system attacks and damages the pancreas to the point where it is unable to produce insulin, the hormone that enables sugar and other nutrients to enter cells. Type 2 diabetes occurs when the body becomes resistant to the effects of insulin. Both disorders lead to high blood sugar levels that, if left untreated, cause numerous complications throughout the body, including the eyes.

People with diabetes are at greater risk of developing cataracts and glaucoma, but a third problem—diabetic retinopathy—is most likely to cause them severe vision loss and blindness. Diabetic retinopathy occurs when high blood sugar levels damage small blood vessels in the retina.

Diabetic retinopathy occurs in two stages. First, the walls of the small blood vessels weaken and leak fluid into the surrounding tissue, often leaving deposits of protein and fat called hard exudates. The vessels also develop microaneurysms, tiny bulges or balloons in their walls that tend to leak red blood cells and plasma into the retina. As the condition progresses, the abnormal vessels begin to close, robbing the retina of its blood supply. Nerve fibers die off because of poor circulation and a lack of oxygen, creating white cottony patches known as soft exudates or cotton-wool spots (see Figure 14, at right).

These changes won't necessarily alter your vision. But if the fluid or blood leakage occurs near the macula—the part of the retina responsible for sharp, central vision—your sight will be impaired (see Figure 15, page 48). When fluid leaks into the center of the macula, the macula can swell, blurring vision. This condition, known as macular edema, can range from minimal to severe.

As retinopathy progresses, the damaged retina tries to repair itself by sprouting new blood vessels. However, these new vessels grow abnormally and extend into the vitreous humor, the gel-filled compartment in front of the retina. The fragile new vessels often leak blood and break. When they bleed into the vitreous humor, they can block the passage of light and cause a sudden loss of vision. The blood is usually reabsorbed, but scar tissue may form. The scar tissue tugs on the retina, pulling it away from the back of the eye, which can lead to permanent vision loss (see "Retinal tear or detachment," page 14). In some cases, the blood does not reabsorb, and surgery may be required to remove the blood and treat the retinopathy.

Figure 14: Diabetic retinopathy

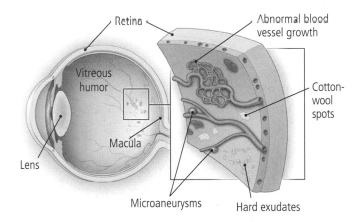

Ongoing high blood sugar levels from poorly managed diabetes can cause the tiny blood vessels in the retina to break down and leak fluid into surrounding tissues, leaving deposits of protein and fat called hard exudates. The vessel walls can also develop tiny bulges called microaneurysms. Eventually, the damage blocks the retina's blood supply. Nerve fibers die, creating white fluffy patches known as cotton-wool spots or soft exudates. New blood vessels may grow, but they are abnormal and often harmful to the retina.

Preventing diabetic retinopathy

One of the best ways to protect your vision if you have diabetes is to control your blood glucose levels. People with diabetes who keep their blood sugar at near-normal levels cut their risk of developing eye diseases and macular edema by 75%. If you have diabetes, also pay careful attention to your blood pressure and cholesterol levels. Above-normal levels increase the likelihood that you'll develop diabetic retinopathy, and that it will significantly affect your vision.

Detecting diabetic retinopathy

The early stages of diabetic retinopathy often have no symptoms. As the damage increases, however, you can develop retinal swelling (macular edema). This can cause a noticeable decline in central vision, especially as the swelling increases.

As diabetic retinopathy advances to its later stage, symptoms become more dramatic. You might notice spots that are really specks of blood floating in your vision. Although sometimes the specks will clear without treatment, you can start to hemorrhage, often while you sleep. Seek immediate treatment from an eye care professional if the specks obscure your vision. Untreated bleeding can become more severe, leading to vision loss and blindness. The sooner you

Figure 15: Diabetic retinopathy vision

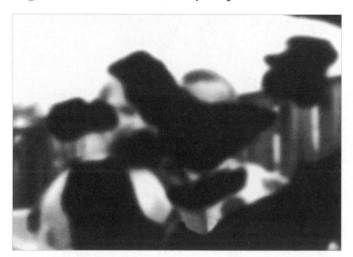

As diabetic retinopathy progresses, you may notice spots and floaters in your vision. Central vision may become distorted.

Photo courtesy of the National Eye Institute.

get help, the better, as earlier treatment is more likely to be effective.

Because diabetic retinopathy often has no early warning signs, the best way to protect yourself is to know whether you're at risk and to get your vision tested as often as necessary. Anyone with diabetes—either type 1 or type 2—should have a comprehensive dilated eye exam at least once a year. Comprehensive eye exams can detect macular edema and even the earliest changes of diabetic retinopathy, including

- leaking blood vessels
- fatty deposits on the retina
- damaged nerve tissue
- microaneurysms.

Prompt treatment can help prevent severe vision loss and blindness.

Treating diabetic retinopathy

There is no cure for diabetic retinopathy, but you can take steps to prevent vision loss—or at least slow its progression. Treatments include laser therapies, anti-VEGF drugs, and steroids. The choice of therapy depends on the type and extent of your retinopathy.

Managing your blood sugar and blood pressure can also slow eye damage and other complications of diabetes. Three other Harvard Special Health Reports—*Living Well with Diabetes*, *Healthy Eating for Type 2 Diabetes*, and *Controlling Your Blood Pressure*—provide more information on these topics. (To order, call 877-649-9457, toll-free, or go online to www. health.harvard.edu.)

Laser treatments

Focal laser treatment is often used for macular edema. In this procedure, the doctor identifies individual leaking blood vessels and seals them off with the laser. This slows leakage and decreases fluid around the retina. Local anesthetics prevent any discomfort during the procedure, which typically involves 20 to 50 laser burns per eye. If macular edema affects both eyes, you'll need a second session—usually a week or so later—for the other eye. The procedure can cut the risk of further vision loss in half, and in a small number of people, it actually restores vision.

Another type of laser procedure, known as scatter laser therapy, is used for advanced retinopathy. The doctor makes 1,000 to 1,500 laser burns in the outer edges of the retina, away from the centrally located macula. Because so many laser burns are needed, treatment may require more than one session. This laser treatment can be uncomfortable, so ask your doctor whether you can get a shot to numb your eye. Scatter laser therapy helps prevent new blood vessel growth. The vessels stop proliferating or even regress, which lowers the risk of hemorrhage or detachment. Possible downsides to this treatment include slight impairments to peripheral vision, color vision, and night vision.

If the bleeding in your eye is severe, you may need to have a vitrectomy before laser surgery. The doctor makes several small incisions in your eye and replaces the vitreous humor (which is clouded with blood) with a salt solution or an air or gas bubble. Your eye will be red and sensitive, and you'll need to use medicated eye drops and wear an eye patch while it heals.

Anti-VEGF drugs

Although laser treatments have been the standard of care for diabetic retinopathy for nearly 30 years, recent research has shown that anti-VEGF drugs—either alone or in combination with laser therapy—may be the best way to prevent vision loss. These drugs, which block a chemical signal that stimulates blood vessel growth, are also used to treat wet AMD (see "Anti-VEGF drugs," page 43).

In April 2017, the FDA approved the anti-VEGF drug ranibizumab (Lucentis) to treat all forms of diabetic retinopathy. The FDA had previously approved Lucentis as a therapy for diabetic macular edema. It's now the only drug that can be used to prevent vision loss in people with all types of diabetic retinopathy. Studies have shown Lucentis improves retinopathy symptoms and slows disease progression significantly more than placebo.

Another anti-VEGF drug, aflibercept (Eylea), is approved only for the treatment of diabetic macular edema. Eylea is currently in a phase 3 trial evaluating it for the treatment of moderately severe to severe diabetic retinopathy without edema. The two-year trial is still ongoing, but at six months, 58% of people treated with Eylea saw greater vision improvements compared with those on placebo. The anti-VEGF cancer drug bevacizumab (Avastin) is also used off-label for diabetic retinopathy.

Another target of drug development is angiopoietin, a family of growth factors that stimulate the development of new blood vessels. Angiopoietin-1 (Ang-1) is essential for the growth of healthy blood vessels. But in people with diabetic eye disease, elevated levels of a related substance—angiopoietin-2 (Ang-2)—lead to leaky, weakened blood vessels. A new drug under investigation, called RG7716, simultaneously blocks Ang-2 and VEGF to protect blood vessels in the eye from damage. Yet another drug under investigation, AKB-9778, acts in a similar way, but on the Tie2 system—a different pathway responsible for healthy blood vessels.

Steroids

Steroid injections have also been used to treat diabetic macular edema. Steroids can reduce retinal swelling and, like anti-VEGF therapies, improve vision for as long as you receive the injections. The benefits often disappear after one to two years, and there are long-term risks, which include the possible development of cataract or glaucoma.

Two steroid implants gradually release steroids into the eye, improving vision for up to three years without the need for injections. Dexamethasone intravitreal implant (Ozurdex) is biodegradable, meaning that it dissolves in the eye and never needs to be removed. It lasts for three or more months. This implant appears less likely to cause glaucoma than traditional steroid injections. The other steroid implant, fluocinolone (Iluvien), can continue to work for up to three years. It also dissolves in the eye, and never needs to be removed. ◆

Living with low vision

More than 25 million people in the United States live with vision that limits their daily activities, a condition known as low vision. Macular degeneration is the most common cause of low vision. Low vision may involve blurry vision, poor central vision, loss of peripheral vision, or even double vision. Whatever the symptom, the immediate consequences are often the same—difficulty performing day-to-day activities such as reading a newspaper, using a computer, watching television, cooking a meal, or crossing the street. Although you may not be able to cure low vision, you often can find ways to cope with it.

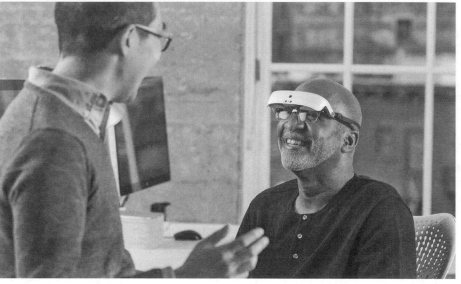

A variety of tools and reading aids can help if you have low vision. For example, electronic low-vision glasses use a high-speed camera and algorithms to digitally enhance images you see.

Magnification tools. The magnifying lens remains one of the most common tools to help compensate for low vision. Most magnifying lenses are handheld, but some are mounted in stands. Others can be incorporated into prescription glass lenses to be used for reading or detail work. Special lenses that work like miniature telescopes can also be mounted on a pair of glasses and used for driving or watching a movie. If you have trouble with excessive glare or reduced contrast (distinction between light and dark), glasses with special filters or stand-mounted magnifiers containing a light source may help.

Electronic low-vision glasses. New technology has opened up a whole new world to people with severe vision loss.

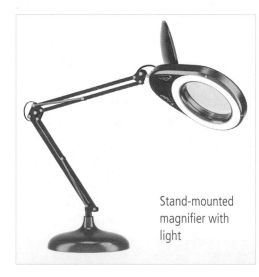

Stand-mounted magnifier with light

Take, for example, eSight—a pair of electronic eyeglasses that uses a high-speed, high-definition camera and computer algorithms to digitally enhance the images you see, in real time. Cutting-edge technology comes with a steep price tag—eSight costs nearly $10,000—but the company has an affordability program to bring these glasses within reach of many consumers.

Computer aids. Many software programs can make the text on a computer monitor larger or more readable. Options include programs that enable you to change font size and background displays, and specialized text-to-speech conversion programs that read text aloud. Separate devices—such as special keyboards or monitor magnifiers—are also available. Most major computer supply stores carry these products.

Reading aids. If you have trouble reading small type, you

Apps for low vision and other eye problems

Cellphones have evolved from devices that can simply make calls to tools that allow you to check email, surf the Internet, schedule your day, and even keep you healthier. A few free or low-cost apps for the iPhone and Android are specifically designed to promote eye health.

Big Clock. If you struggle to see the numbers on your clock, this large-numbered phone app makes it much easier for you to tell time.

Eye Drops Alarm. This free iPhone app reminds you when to take your eye drops after surgery, or if you have a condition like glaucoma or dry eye. It even tells you the bottle cap color and in which eye to insert the drops.

EyeXam. This app lets you test your vision, which can help you determine whether it's time for a checkup with your ophthalmologist. EyeXam also will help you locate an eye doctor in your area and schedule an appointment.

i-Read, Smart Magnifier, and Magnifying Glass with Light. These apps turn your iPhone or Android phone into a magnifying glass and light, making it easier to read menus in dimly lit restaurants or programs in dark theaters.

MaculaTester. This interactive version of the Amsler grid not only helps you identify vision changes that can signal macular degeneration or retinopathy, but also allows you to record the area where you notice distortion so you can share the information with your ophthalmologist.

---

can buy any number of assistive products. Inexpensive, low-tech vision aids include large-print versions of address books, checks, utility bills, playing cards, and phones. "Talking" watches, alarm clocks, pillboxes, and calculators allow you to hear, rather than see, numbers and words. Video magnifiers project the words from a book or other reading material onto a large screen. And smart speakers like the Amazon Echo and Google Home let you call up information instantly using voice commands ("Alexa, what will the weather be like tomorrow?").

Another option is to buy large-print versions of newspapers and books. Or, purchase an e-reader like the Kindle or Nook, which increase word size, improve contrast, and sometimes provide a light source to enhance readability and reduce eyestrain. Audiobooks provide yet another alternative, and you can conveniently download them to your smartphone. Speaking of which, many smartphones come complete with virtual assistants (like Siri) who will respond to your voice queries and commands, much like smart speakers do. Smartphones and tablets also come with large-sized print options and adjustable lighting. And, you can purchase special apps for people with low vision, such as EyeNote, which reads the denominations of money for you.

You can order many low-vision devices through several organizations, including the Low Vision Center (see "Resources," page 52).

Improved lighting. By age 60, your retina requires three times as much light as it did when you were 20. One very easy way to see more clearly is to improve the lighting in your home. Use brighter bulbs. Position lamps so that the light shines directly onto the materials in front of you. Choosing a light with an adjustable neck can help you focus the beam right where you need it.

Adaptation. In addition to using various gadgets, you can learn a few simple tricks to compensate for diminished sight and make your home safer.

- Arrange furniture so you have a clear path to walk, and reduce clutter in your home to prevent falls.
- Remove or tape down throw rugs.
- Buy plates and cups in colors that contrast with your tablecloth or placemats.
- Label your foods and medications with large print (Sharpie pens are useful for this) to make them easier to identify.

Ophthalmologists, optometrists, and occupational therapists can help you learn these and other techniques.

Whatever your vision problem, there are now more ways to cope with it than ever before. But remember, regardless of your age, the single most important thing you can do is to have your eyes checked regularly and follow your doctor's treatment recommendations. By doing that and following the simple steps outlined in this report, you can protect your eyes and help preserve your vision as you age. ♥

Resources

Organizations

American Academy of Ophthalmology
655 Beach St.
San Francisco, CA 94109
415-561-8500
www.aao.org/eye-health

The American Academy of Ophthalmology is the world's largest association of eye doctors and surgeons. Its EyeSmart website offers eye disease prevention tips, a guide to common eye conditions and their symptoms, and specific answers about eye diseases from ophthalmologists.

American Glaucoma Society
655 Beach St.
San Francisco, CA 94109
415-561-8587
www.americanglaucomasociety.net

This organization of glaucoma specialists is committed to providing top-quality care and education to people with this eye disease. On its website, the society offers patient-focused educational materials about glaucoma diagnosis and treatment.

American Macular Degeneration Foundation
P.O. Box 515
Northampton, MA 01061
413-268-7660
www.macular.org

This nonprofit supports scientific research on AMD and provides information and support for patients and their families.

EyeCare America
P.O. Box 429098
San Francisco, CA 94142
877-887-6327 (toll-free)
www.aao.org/eyecare-america

This program of the American Academy of Ophthalmology offers eye exams and medication assistance.

Glaucoma Research Foundation
251 Post St., Suite 600
San Francisco, CA 94108
800-826-6693 (toll-free)
www.glaucoma.org

This foundation provides educational materials on glaucoma and publishes a free newsletter, *Gleams*, three times a year.

Lighthouse Guild
250 W. 64th St.
New York, NY 10023
800-284-4422 (toll-free)
www.lighthouseguild.org

Lighthouse provides educational materials on age-related vision problems and offers referrals to vision and rehabilitation agencies. Call for a catalog of aids for daily living.

Low Vision Center
4905 Del Ray Ave., Suite 504
Bethesda, MD 20814
301-951-4444
www.lowvisioninfo.org

The center offers information to help people with limited vision remain independent and lead fuller lives.

National Eye Institute
Information Office
31 Center Drive, MSC 2510
Bethesda, MD 20892
301-496-5248
www.nei.nih.gov

Part of the National Institutes of Health, the National Eye Institute provides up-to-date information on eye diseases and research.

Prevent Blindness
211 W. Wacker Drive, Suite 1700
Chicago, IL 60606
800-331-2020 (toll-free)
www.preventblindness.org

Prevent Blindness provides fact sheets, brochures, and other informational material on eye safety, eye care, vision screening, and eye ailments.

Harvard Special Health Reports

The following reports from Harvard Medical School go into greater detail on various topics mentioned in this report. You can order them by going online to www.health.harvard.edu or calling 877-649-9457 (toll-free).

Controlling Your Blood Pressure: What to do when your doctor says you have hypertension
Randall M. Zusman, M.D., Medical Editor
(Harvard Medical School, 2018)

This report explains how to keep blood pressure in a healthy range by making lifestyle changes, such as losing weight, increasing activity, and eating more healthfully. A Special Section includes 20 strategies for cutting back on salt. The report also explains the many types of blood pressure medications.

Healthy Eating for Type 2 Diabetes
David M. Nathan, M.D., and Linda Delahanty, M.S., R.D., L.D.N., Medical Editors
(Harvard Medical School, 2012)

This report describes the components of a healthy diet for people with diabetes as well as how to work with a dietitian, develop a meal plan, fit physical activity into your schedule, and make wise choices dining out, all while staying on track with losing weight.

Living Well with Diabetes: Smart strategies for controlling your blood sugar
David M. Nathan, M.D., Medical Editor
(Harvard Medical School, 2018)

This report describes the biology of diabetes and includes detailed information on strategies, from medications to lifestyle changes, that help control blood sugar. It explains how and when to monitor your blood sugar and how to cope with both short- and long-term complications of the disease.

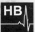 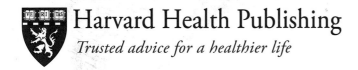

Harvard Health Publishing
Trusted advice for a healthier life

 **Receive *HEALTHbeat*, Harvard Health Publishing's free email newsletter**

Go to: **www.health.harvard.edu** to subscribe to *HEALTHbeat*. This free weekly email newsletter brings you health tips, advice, and information on a wide range of topics.

You can also join in discussion with experts from Harvard Health Publishing and folks like you on a variety of health topics, medical news, and views by reading the Harvard Health Blog (**www.health.harvard.edu/blog**).

Order this report and other publications from Harvard Medical School

online | **www.health.harvard.edu**

phone | **877-649-9457** (toll-free)

mail | **Belvoir Media Group**
Attn: Harvard Health Publishing
P.O. Box 5656
Norwalk, CT 06856-5656

Licensing, bulk rates, or corporate sales

email | **HHP_licensing@hms.harvard.edu**

online | **www.content.health.harvard.edu**

Other publications from Harvard Medical School

Special Health Reports *Harvard Medical School publishes in-depth reports on a wide range of health topics, including:*

Addiction	Eye Disease	Pain Relief
Allergies	Foot Care	Positive Psychology
Advance Care Planning	Grief & Loss	Prostate Disease
Alzheimer's Disease	Hands	Reducing Sugar & Salt
Anxiety & Stress Disorders	Headache	Rheumatoid Arthritis
Back Pain	Hearing Loss	Sensitive Gut
Balance	Heart Disease	Sexuality
Caregiving	Heart Disease & Diet	Skin Care
Change Made Easy	Heart Failure	Sleep
Cholesterol	High Blood Pressure	Strength Training
Cognitive Fitness	Incontinence	Stress Management
COPD	Knees & Hips	Stretching
Core Workout	Life After Cancer	Stroke
Depression	Living Longer	Tai Chi
Diabetes	Memory	Thyroid Disease
Diabetes & Diet	Men's Health	Vitamins & Minerals
Energy/Fatigue	Neck Pain	Walking for Health
Erectile Dysfunction	Nutrition	Weight Loss
Exercise	Osteoarthritis	Women's Health
Exercise Your Joints	Osteoporosis	Yoga

Periodicals *Monthly newsletters and annual publications, including:*

Harvard Health Letter	*Harvard Heart Letter*	*Prostate Disease Annual*
Harvard Women's Health Watch	*Harvard Men's Health Watch*	

ISBN 978-1-61401-201-6

ISBN 978-1-61401-201-6
SX20000

AE11

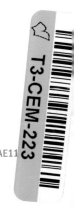

Glossary

accommodation: The ability of the eye's lens to focus at a range of distances.

age-related macular degeneration (AMD): A condition, more common with age, characterized by damage to the macula—an area in the center of the retina that's responsible for producing clear vision.

anterior chamber: The space behind the cornea and in front of the iris; it is filled with aqueous humor.

aqueous humor: The watery fluid that nourishes the eye and fills the anterior and posterior chambers.

astigmatism: A refractive error characterized by irregular curvature of the cornea, causing distorted images.

cataract: A clouding of the previously clear lens of the eye, which is typically associated with aging.

cones: Specialized cells in the retina that are sensitive to color and light; they are more active in light than in darkness, provide sharp vision, and are abundant in the macular area of the retina.

conjunctiva: The transparent membrane that lines the eyelid and covers the front portion of the sclera.

conjunctivitis: Swelling of the conjunctiva due to an infection or irritants in the environment. Also called "pink eye."

cornea: The curved, transparent dome of tissue at the front of the eye, through which light first passes on its way into the eye.

diabetic retinopathy: A diabetes complication caused by damage to blood vessels in the retina.

drusen: Tiny yellow deposits that form beneath the macula and may indicate the early stages of age-related macular degeneration.

farsightedness: A type of refractive error in which distant objects appear clear, but close ones appear blurry (see also hyperopia).

flashes: Streaks or flashes of light in the field of vision, caused by changes to the vitreous humor.

floaters: Specks or other shapes that float across the field of vision, caused by shrinkage of the vitreous humor.

fluorescein angiography: A diagnostic test that photographs blood vessels in the retina after the intravenous injection of a special dye.

fovea: A pit-like area in the middle of the macula that provides the clearest vision.

glaucoma: A collection of diseases that damage the eye's optic nerve, sometimes to the point of severe vision loss or blindness.

hyperopia: An optical error in which light rays reach the retina before converging at a focal point; commonly known as farsightedness.

intraocular lens: A small artificial lens permanently fixed inside the eye to replace the natural lens during cataract surgery.

iris: The colored ring in front of the lens that controls the size of the pupil and how much light enters the eye.

lacrimal gland: The gland that produces tears. It is located in the upper, outer section of the eye's orbit.

lens: A flexible, transparent structure directly behind the iris that focuses rays of light onto the retina.

macula: The area of the retina packed with cones, which is responsible for sharp central vision.

myopia: An optical error in which light rays meet and focus before reaching the retina; also known as nearsightedness.

nearsightedness: A type of refractive error in which close objects appear clear, but distant objects appear blurry (see also myopia).

ophthalmoscope: An instrument with a light and mirrors for examining the deep interior of the eye.

optic nerve: A "cable" that emanates from the back of the eye, consisting of specialized nerve fibers that transmit visual impulses to the brain.

orbit: The bony socket that surrounds the eyeball.

peripheral vision: Side vision, or what the eye perceives outside the direct line of vision.

posterior chamber: The area behind the iris and in front of the lens that is filled with aqueous humor.

presbyopia: An age-related condition that prevents the eye from focusing clearly on objects up close.

retina: The innermost layer of the eye, consisting of specialized cells and lining nearly three-quarters of the back of the eye. It converts light energy to electrical energy and sends visual images to the brain via the optic nerve.

rods: Light-sensitive cells in the retina that respond best in darkness and dim light.

Schlemm's canal: A channel through which fluid drains from the trabecular meshwork into the bloodstream.

sclera: The white of the eye. This tough, protective coating of collagen and elastic tissue, together with the cornea, makes up the outer layer of the eyeball.

slit lamp: An instrument that magnifies internal structures of the eye with the aid of a beam of light directed through a narrow slit.

tonometry: A glaucoma screening test that measures pressure inside the eye.

trabecular meshwork: A structure through which fluid drains out of the eye. Problems with the trabecular meshwork can cause fluid to build up and eye pressure to increase.

visual acuity: The eye's ability to see sharply. Acuity is usually measured in comparison with what a normal eye would see from 20 feet.

visual field: The scope of what the eye sees, including central and peripheral vision.

vitreous humor: The clear, gel-like substance that fills the space behind the lens and supports the shape of the rear portion of the eye.